# Peer Supervision Groups

# Peer Supervision Groups

## *How They Work and Why You Need One*

Lee D. Kassan

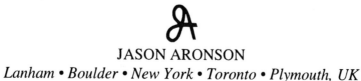

JASON ARONSON

*Lanham • Boulder • New York • Toronto • Plymouth, UK*

Published by Jason Aronson
An imprint of Rowman & Littlefield Publishers, Inc.
A wholly owned subsidiary of The Rowman & Littlefield Publishing Group, Inc.
4501 Forbes Boulevard, Suite 200, Lanham, Maryland 20706
www.rowmanlittlefield.com

Estover Road, Plymouth PL6 7PY, United Kingdom

British Library Cataloguing in Publication Information Available

**Library of Congress Cataloging-in-Publication Data**
Kassan, Lee D.
  Peer supervision groups : how they work and why you need one / Lee D. Kassan.
    p. ; cm.
  Includes bibliographical references and index.
  ISBN 978-0-7657-0696-6
  1. Peer review in psychiatry. 2. Psychiatrists—Supervision of. I. Title.
  [DNLM: 1. Peer Group. 2. Psychotherapy—methods. 3. Education, Medical,
Continuing—organization & administration. 4. Interprofessional Relations. WM 21]
  RC455.2.P43.K37 2010
  616.890068—dc22                                                    2010032849

Printed in the United States of America

# Contents

# Introduction

What is a peer supervision group, and why would anyone want to belong to one? The name is pretty much self-explanatory. It is a group of professionals, clinicians and practitioners, who meet regularly as a group to give feedback and supervision to each other. For many clinicians, especially those in private practice, membership in a peer supervision group is an essential part of their professional lives, as it has been of mine. Yet very little has been written about these groups. This book will examine the subject in depth. While there have been several articles about peer supervision groups, which we shall review in some detail in Chapters 1 and 2, there has never been a book devoted specifically to this important topic. This book tries to fill that gap.

Some of the few authors who have tackled the subject in articles have given working definitions of the peer group. Goldberg (1981) describes it as "an opportunity for exchange with trusted colleagues, for the evocation of deeply encountered feelings about their work and the processes and directions toward which they aspire as purposive beings" (p. 27). Counselman and Weber (2004) describe it as a group that "meets[s] regularly to discuss cases and other professional matters" (p. 125). Counselman and Weber go on to specify several purposes, including "ongoing support and consultation for difficult cases; combating the isolation and potential burnout inherent in psychotherapy practice; and offering important networking, marketing, and other professional development opportunities" (p. 125–126).

Although they accept the usual name for such groups, Counselman and Weber (2004) point out that technically these are *consultation* groups, not supervision groups, since, according to the definition they use, *supervision* implies a power differential, and a supervisor often has some responsibility for the patient. As we shall see, this issue of the power of the supervisor is often one of the reasons experienced clinicians seek out a peer group situation rather than a conventional supervision arrangement.

I think my own experience in supervision is fairly typical. I trained and got my certification in psychotherapy and psychoanalysis at the American Institute for Psychotherapy and Psychoanalysis in New York City between 1978 and 1984. In addition to course work, four years of supervision and one year of case control (in which the trainee and supervisor follow a single patient for the entire year) were required. While I have discussed at greater length my experience in supervision elsewhere (Kassan, 1996), I will say briefly here that my supervisors ranged from very good to disappointing. We often butted heads on what was best for the patient, and I can remember often withholding something I thought the supervisor would object to or criticize (see Chapter 2: The Problems of Supervision). I think I have learned more from my peer group than I ever did from my supervisors and with less conflict, less shame, and less defensiveness.

Having been in one peer supervision group or another since the beginning of my professional career over thirty years ago, I know how important having the support of the group has been for me. I have met many other colleagues who have been in groups of their own, often for many years. I hope that this book will inspire those professionals not in peer groups now to want to join one, or even to start their own.

When I ask people who are not in a peer group why they're not, the answers fall into two categories: "I'm too busy," and "I can't find one." I'm skeptical of both these explanations. I think that many people are afraid to present their work, and use these reasons as excuses. Billow and Mendelsohn (1987) appear to agree. They suggest that "avoidant feelings, involving . . . essentially paranoid dynamics, conflict with approach needs. These include fantasies of shame, humiliation, contempt, rejection, and fears of exposure, ridicule, abandonment, ostracism, censure, etc." (pp. 36–37). They also point out that, because peers are chosen for "benefits beyond mere friendship" (p. 37), including referrals, consultant positions, and enhanced professional status, the question arises of whether one will "risk being truly open when reputation and position are at stake" (p. 37). I hope that, after reading this book, clinicians will find some way to overcome these resistances and seek out a peer group. Two hours or less every other week seems achievable for everyone, especially when it is clearly this important, and there are many groups available. If you can't find one, why not start one? I believe it is too important to do without.

The book is divided into four parts. In Part I, I look closely at supervision: in general, in groups, and in peer groups, and examine some of the problems of the supervisory relationship. In Part II, I present the responses of thirty-four members of twenty different peer supervision groups, and look at all aspects of peer group functioning. I will briefly describe and compare my own experience after each question, and then discuss the issues more objectively at the end of each chapter. In Part III, I describe nine different peer groups, one at length (my own group) in fairly deep detail. In the last part, I will spell out very specific recommendations for organizing and running a peer group.

In general, I prefer to write about topics that I believe have been neglected in the literature (Kassan, 1996, 1999, 2007, 2008). Peer supervision groups are an important part of so many therapists' lives, yet so little has been written on the topic. I have wanted to address this topic for a while, and was finally able to do so. I want to thank all the peer group members who agreed to be interviewed and shared their experiences with me. Although they must remain anonymous, I want them to know how grateful I am. I could not have done this book without them. I'd like to thank my editor, Julie Kirsch, for her wise suggestions for improving the book. I would also like to thank L. M. M., my partner in life, for love, support, and thoughtful input on the manuscript.

# Part I

# Supervision

# Chapter 1

# The Supervisory Relationship

Supervision has been a significant part of training in psychotherapy from the birth of the profession. Freud himself had his Wednesday circle, where cases were presented and feedback was given (Nunberg & Federa, 1962). Most authorities make it quite clear that they consider supervision an essential component of training.

Alonso (1985), in one of the more well-known books about supervision, tries to define the word, starting with the literature from the Berlin Psychoanalytic Institute. She says that supervision is seen in three different ways: "1) a cognitive and primarily didactic process; 2) an emotional growth experience for the maturing clinician; and 3) an interpersonal process that focuses on the empathic connectedness between the concerned parties" (p. 13). If the supervisor uses the first definition, he or she will take the position that "any difficulties in the supervisory situation can be understood as a problem of insufficient data due to incomplete or poor teaching, or as an inability on the part of the trainee to understand, recall, or apply theory to technique, and so forth" (p. 15). Someone who uses the second definition will "assume that the development of a clinician from novice to expert is primarily an emotional, maturational process, much like the development of a child from infancy to adulthood" (p. 17). She adds that this kind of supervisor "is clearly focused on the clinician first, and on the patient secondarily" (p. 19). Alonso sees the third definition as a middle position that combines elements of both. Alonso recommends that beginning supervisors have formal training, including presentation of a supervisory session to a group for feedback.

In her book, Alonso (1985) examines supervision primarily in an institutional setting, whereas many people seek supervision even when they are finished with their basic training. Hess (1986), in his review of

7

Alonso, finds the book a little naïve, suggesting that Alonso tends to idealize the supervisor, and says "it offers a good summary of dynamic supervision but does not offer any empirical support for its assertions, nor does it offer serious reflection concerning its theoretical claims" (p. 1005). Pines (1987) says of Alonso that "her perspective reflects the North American context, and is therefore not always applicable elsewhere; however, there is much that speaks directly to all our experience" (p. 381). Pines finds that she avoids discussion of more difficult patients and, by extension, of more difficult supervisory relationships and interactions.

In their study, Tyler, Sloan, and King (2000) found that "[a]lthough there was individual difference variability, results suggest that the typical full-time faculty supervisor spends nearly seven hours per week conducting individual and group supervision and is responsible for four graduate trainees, each of whom carry four cases. Typically, case discussion is used considerably more than are other modalities, such as listening to audiotapes, viewing videotapes, and conducting live supervision. The typical supervisee receives about two and a half hours of supervision per week through some combination of individual and group mentoring" (p. 100). They also found that "[d]espite devoting over six hours per week to supervisory duties and their attendant stresses and liabilities, half of our respondents reported no additional compensation beyond their regular salaries. Given that in many academic settings supervisory activities receive little weight in promotion and tenure considerations, this finding is consistent with concerns that clinical supervision is often undervalued in academia" (p. 101). These findings suggest that, at least in many institutional settings, supervision is relatively less important than other aspects of training.

## Individual supervision

An individual trainee with an individual supervisor is considered essential in the beginning stages of training by most writers on the subject. Pate and Wolff (1990) identified three factors as the most important elements of satisfactory supervision: the supervisor's teaching ability, rapport between the supervisor and the trainee, and the supervisor's fund of knowledge. Lachmann (2003) says the supervision is a complicated endeavor and that "balance needs to be maintained between too dogged attention to details, which can lead the supervisee to feel outclassed, criticized, shamed, and constricted, on one hand, and abandoned and deprived of support because of insufficient input, on the other" (p. 342).

In their survey, Hess and Hess (1983) found that, even though they were untrained in supervision, most supervisors did a decent job. In their study, "[s]upervisors had 9.3 years of clinical experience and 7.6 years of supervisory experience. Yet they apparently lack training in psychotherapy supervision, given that only one third of the facilities reported training for supervisors. Perhaps the assumption is made that the clinicians were already trained when hired for the position, that they would learn to supervise on the job, that being a therapist is sufficient supervisory training, or that having been supervised imparts supervision training. These assumptions are questionable, since few doctoral programs . . . or internships offer supervisory training" (pp. 511–512). In spite of these realities, Hess and Hess found that "[i]n summary, supervisors tend to be well trained, moderately experienced, and professionally committed to supervision, although untrained in supervision specifically" (p. 512).

Overholser (2004) reminds us that protecting the client is also an important component of supervision, especially with neophyte therapists. He proposes a model of "four pillars" that includes developing a positive working alliance, providing directive guidance, using a Socratic dialogue to explore key issues, and customizing the supervision to match the needs of the trainee. Overholser (1991, 2004) advocates a supervisory approach that uses the Socratic method of asking questions because "explicit instructions can be counterproductive" (p. 68) and that "more insight is attained when people discover a relationship on their own than when it is explained to them" (p. 68). According to Overholser, this kind of supervision is more effective because it "helps supervisees to learn the processes involved in psychotherapy instead of simply imitating what they have observed" (p. 68). In ideal circumstances, "the Socratic supervisor functions not as a lecturer, but as a catalyst, forcing supervisees to realize that the answers lie within themselves" (p. 68). The peer supervision group is more consistent with this model than the usual kind of supervision.

Similarly, Rabinowitz, Heppner, and Roehlke (1986) found "that a sense of security and support between supervisor and supervisee is necessary in the beginning stage of supervision" (p. 298), and that "trainees from a more advanced level were more open to examining personal issues in supervision" (p. 299). Crick (1991) discusses her own experience and finds that the very nature of supervision puts the trainee in an adolescent position. Crick found that supervisors who respect the supervisee and use a dialectic rather than a didactic style were preferred. Shanfield, Mohl, Matthews, and Hetherly (1992) found that the most important characteristics in highly rated supervisors were empathy, an experiential orientation, focus on the therapist, some didactic features (clarification and interpretation), and the depth to which they explored an issue.

Allen, Szollos, and Williams (1986) found that "[g]ood supervisors modeled respect of both their and their trainees' differences in values, experiences, and personal privacy. From this nonintrusive and pluralistic base, they provided useful, theory-based conceptual frameworks for understanding psychotherapeutic processes; taught practical skills; and encouraged trainees to experiment with using novel strategies. Good supervisors also were tolerant of mistakes, provided clear and direct feedback, and confronted supervisees' resistances in an atmosphere of safety. They also invested more time in the process and monitored the psychotherapeutic activities of their charges by some means other than trainees' self-reports. Finally, they were open to feedback about their own styles of relating" (p. 97).

In their small survey, Worthen and McNeill (1996) explored the experience of "good" supervision events from the perspective of the supervisees. Eight intermediate-level to advanced-level trainees described a recent good supervision experience, and these were qualitatively analyzed. They identified four distinct supervision phases: (a) existential baseline, (b) setting the stage, (c) good supervision experience, and (d) outcomes of good supervision. The quality of the supervisory relationship was cited as a crucial and pivotal component by all supervisees. "In each of the eight transcripts examined, participants referred to the quality of the supervisory relationship as crucial and pivotal. Perhaps over the course of an entire semester of supervision, the supervisory relationship, although a significant factor in supervision, would not always play a predominant part in each session, and other issues might become more focal. However, it is likely that, in the course of addressing the variety of supervision issues, the supervisory relationship would continue to serve as the base of all good therapeutic and professional training, suggesting that the learning and acquisition of professional skills and identity may be delayed, hampered, or not fully developed outside the context of an effective supervisory relationship" (p. 32).

In addition, Worthen and McNeill found that "[w]ithin this structure, many of the themes and events are also generally consistent with previous quantitative studies in terms of what constitutes good supervision. For example, events reflected positive aspects of the supervisory relationship, which include supervisor self-disclosure . . . as experienced by participants in this study as a technique helpful in normalizing the struggle, a supervisory environment of experimentation and acceptance of mistakes and failures . . . task orientations specific to developmental level . . . and expression of warmth be the ability to perceive therapeutic activities with an increased comprehensiveness and sophistication" (p. 32).

In another study, Murray (1974) measured attitudes toward supervision and supervisors and found that for most supervision was viewed as a positive experience, "although it was felt by both faculty (83 percent) and students (73 percent) that supervision was not all that it could be as a learning experience" (p. 293). For example, "[n]inety percent of the faculty felt that the evaluation of students was based upon the student's ability, but 50 percent of the students believe that their marks were based more on their personalities than on their abilities" (p. 293).

Yerushalmi (1992a) draws a parallel between the developing child and the developing therapist and suggests that in supervision "there should be quite a few moments in which the supervisor, like the mother, does not intervene, and is silent but attentive" (p. 263). Otherwise the therapist in training may form a *false self* (Winnicott, 1965). This situation may create a conflict for the supervisor between the developmental needs of the supervisee and the therapeutic needs of the patient. In a similar vein, Yerushalmi (1999b) proposes that both supervisor and supervisee "play" in the supervisory sessions as a way of understanding what is going on in therapy with the patient, although he acknowledges that this is almost impossible in the current climate of managed care and evidence-based treatment. Yerushalmi (1994) also suggests that the model of self psychology is a useful one for the supervision situation, so that supervisors provide an atmosphere of acceptance. Empathic failures by the supervisor need the same examination and working through that they do in the therapy situation. Steinhelber, Patterson, Cliffe, and Le-Goullon (1984) found that there was no correlation between patient improvement and the amount of supervision the therapist had, but did find that patients showed significant improvement when the therapist and the supervisor shared similar theoretical orientations.

In their research review, Allen, Szollos, and Williams (1986 found that "[s]tudies that assess specific supervisory practices generally indicate that supervisees are satisfied with their experiences. Literature dealing more generally with training practices in clinical and counseling psychology, however, suggests the existence of greater dissatisfaction" (p. 91). They found that the "best and worst experiences could be differentiated most strongly by perceived expertise and trustworthiness of the supervisor" (p. 95). Their conclusions were that "greater satisfaction with supervision is determined more by supervisors' general assumptive, theoretical, and stylistic stances than by how training is structured or how particular interventions are used. The existence of a supportive relationship is frequently cited as the essential ingredient of successful supervision" (p. 97).

Cresci (1996) found that ratings of supervisory sessions and the amount learned in them varied greatly, depending on who was doing the rating: the supervisor or the trainee. Supervisees rate sessions more positively when they are less anxious, and she advises supervisors to monitor the anxiety level of the trainee carefully. Shanfield, Matthews, & Hetherly (1993) found that supervisors with the highest ratings were the ones who consistently addressed the trainees' anxieties and issues, rather than following their own agendas. Supervisors with low ratings paid little or no attention to the resident's issues. Emerson (1996) also found that it is crucial to reduce fear and anxiety for learning to take place.

Webb and Wheeler (1998) found that "supervisees were likely to disclose more in individual rather than in collective supervision, when their supervisor was someone whom they themselves had chosen rather than had allocated to them, and when they were supervised independently of the setting in which they counseled rather than in-house. There was a positive correlation between the quality of the supervisory working alliance as experienced by the supervisee and the extent of his or her disclosure" (p. 522).

In a survey of forty-eight trainees, twelve each from clinical psychology, counseling psychology, psychiatry, and social work, Nelson (1978) found that supervisees were most interested in gaining therapeutic competence, and that their ideal way of acquiring this was by direct observation of the supervisor conducting therapy, either on videotape or live behind a one-way mirror. (I know of very few people who had this in his or her training; I myself never did in six years of supervision.) "Since helping trainees gain therapeutic competence is clearly the chief purpose for providing formal training in psychotherapy, it is logical that trainees would prefer supervisory methods that provide the supervisor with a maximum amount of information regarding trainee therapy sessions (e.g., videotaping or direct observation) and that provide trainees with actual demonstrations of appropriate therapy techniques (e.g., direct observation of the supervisor conducting therapy)" (p. 547). Subjects in Nelson's study reported that the most desirable supervisors would be flexible, self-revealing, permissive, and outgoing. "In view of the complexity of the psychotherapeutic process and the variety of theories to which trainees are typically exposed, it is reasonable that trainees would prefer flexible, permissive supervisors who encourage experimentation with various approaches and allow each trainee to develop an individualized therapeutic style" (p. 547). *yes.*

There is a controversy about what approach makes for the best and most thorough supervisory experience: Is supervision exclusively a didactic approach, or should it also explore the trainee's intrapsychic issues, as in psychotherapy? Itzhaky & Itzhaky (1996) have some suggestions for helping the supervisor avoid crossing the line into therapy. Cohen and DeBetz (1977) define the supervisory relationship and state quite clearly that it is not psychotherapy of the trainee. Counselman and Gumpert (1993) and Moss (1995) make a clear division between supervision and therapy for the therapist in training. Both papers emphasize the importance of a clear and specific contract with the supervisor that draws these boundaries.

On the other hand, Langs (1994) suggests the best supervisory experience occurs within the framework of a comparable form of therapy. Montgomery (1978) suggests that, because all the different therapeutic approaches seem to have the same effectiveness, it is less important for the supervisor to focus on didactic material and more useful to model what a good therapist does by listening and asking questions. She takes the side that it is part of the supervisor's job to help the trainee work through personal issues by both modeling and by being available as therapist if necessary. Hunt (1981) suggests that discussion and analysis of countertransference should be part of the supervisory session, if the supervisor maintains a readiness to seek the origins of the countertransference emotions in the therapist's interaction with the patient. In his article, Hirsch (1998) comments on the articles by Frawley-O'Dea (1998) and by Sarnat (1998). Frawley-O'Dea examines the interplay between a supervisee's personal analysis and his or her supervision. Sarnat attempts to make the case for the value of acknowledging and working with regressive phenomena that arise within the supervisory relationship. And Hirsch agrees with both Frawley-O'Dea's and Sarnat's position that the examination of both countertransference and affective engagement in the supervisory relationship is important and sometimes necessary.

## Group Supervision

Group supervision means several trainees with a single supervisor. The advantages of group supervision are several: the trainee gets multiple points of view, from both the supervisor and the other supervisees, maximizing opportunities for learning; the trainee has the opportunity to watch others present cases, which can reduce shame and self-criticism; and the trainee can feel the support of the other group members, making it easier to challenge the authority of the supervisor.

Ogren, Apelman, and Klawitter (2001) and Ogren and Sundin (2007) strongly endorse the use of group supervision, although they acknowledge that the theoretical advantages and the actual situations may be very different. Mintz (1983) argues that group supervision offers more advantages than the traditional supervisory dyad because trainees benefit from hearing the self-doubt and insecurity of their peers. Group supervision also offers a buffer against an authoritarian or abusive supervisor (see Chapter 2). Ettin (1995) says that group supervision of group therapy, in a consultation group structure, can be very helpful as the parallel process in the consultation group illuminates the problem in the presenter's therapy group. Aronson (1990) finds that the goals of group supervision are the same as individual supervision, but that more and possibly better insights may be expected from the group than from a single supervisor, and these insights are more likely to occur if the leader and the group members all believe that others' points of view are valuable and deserve consideration.

Moss (1995) finds that group supervision allows trainees to listen without as much anxiety as in individual supervision, and that other members may be able to help if an impasse arises between the supervisor and a trainee. He advocates a focus on countertransference issues, which may be more easily illuminated by the parallel process that can occur in group supervision of therapy groups. Altfeld and Bernard (1999) also discuss the advantages of supervising group therapists in a group setting. Parallel processes in the supervisory group can illuminate the dynamics of the therapy group being presented. Rosenthal (2005) also advocates group supervision for group therapists. He believes that supervision in a group helps the budding group therapist to think in terms of group dynamics rather than as a collection of individuals.

In separate reviews of the literature on group supervision, Holloway and Johnston (1985), and later Prieto (1996), found that there was little if any actual research on the subject, and that groups were structured on intuitive, commonsense principles. Enyedy and colleagues (2003) refer to these articles in doing their own study of group supervision. "In 1985, Holloway and Johnston demonstrated just how little research was available to support this common supervision format. In a later follow-up, Prieto (1996) found that little had changed with respect to research on group supervision during the intervening decade. Most of the group supervision literature, therefore, remains either conceptual or based on practitioner observations" (p. 312). Their own study found that problems clustered in five main areas: between-member problems, including competition, conflict, and member nonparticipation; problems with the supervisor, including negative behaviors or lack of experience; supervisee anxiety and other negative feelings; logistical problems, such as room size and session schedule; and poor group time management. They seemed to think that most if not all of these problems were remediable by a well-trained and effective group leader.

Counselman and Gumpert (1993) say that group supervision can be very useful and effective, and has some advantages over individual supervision for more experienced therapists, but not for beginners. They divide these advantages into *case-related* and *therapist-related* categories. Case-related advantages include "a wider array of perspectives and strategies" (p. 26) and the greater likelihood that parallel process in the group will reveal more about the case. The group can offer more compelling feedback than an individual supervisor. "It is harder to argue with an observation or interpretation made by four or five therapists than by one" (p. 27). Therapist-related advantages include the community and support of the group. Most clinicians in private practice easily get isolated. "A supervision group provides a place not only to continue to learn, but also to let off steam, share one's anxieties and insecurities, laugh, cry, and generally be with other professionals who care about each other and share concerns about the work" (p. 27).

Advocating group supervision as part of training of supervisors, Yerushalmi (1999a) notes that "there have been few efforts to study the process of supervision of supervision or to understand its nature and what makes it work" (p. 427). He suggests that doing supervision is part of a lifelong learning process. He recommends that group supervision of supervision itself be an integral part of the curriculum of any senior professional who is involved in regular supervision of trainees. "As senior professionals, for whom therapeutic work and functioning are central constituents of self-image, participants in the supervisors' group need to remind themselves that professional development never ends. Substantial investment in the group and establishment of a work team that upholds ethical principles and allows its members to bring themselves as completely and authentically as possible to their supervisory work contribute to the participants' professional development, advance their growth as supervisors, and play an important role in the evolution of the organization that they serve. Notwithstanding all the potential problems mentioned above, group supervision of supervision is highly recommended as a professional activity for psychoanalytically oriented training programs and, as such, deserves a great deal of theoretical and organizational attention. It is potentially an undertaking that furthers professional and personal development at all levels of training programs" (p. 445).

Yerushalmi (1999a) believes that group supervision can help prevent burnout. "In my opinion, meetings of this kind, which offer supervisors guidance in their supervisory functioning, provide an important counterbalance to the feelings of depletion and exhaustion that may plague the experienced supervisor who is faced with an ongoing flow of complex supervisory issues" (p. 428). This does not mean that there are no problems, however, and there may be darker undercurrents that must be addressed. "I propose that because the members of a supervisors' group are at the same stage of professional development and have a similar professional status, they are in a competitive situation. Besides the support, holding, and sense of similarity that the other members of the group provide for each of the participants, there is also competition for recognition, admiration of one's professional methods, and power. When all these can be expressed appropriately and moderately, they confirm the supervisors' feelings of validity, self-assertiveness, and ability to influence their environment. It is particularly important for supervision-of-supervision groups that these two elements should be combined" (Yerushalmi, 1999a, p. 436).

## Peer Supervision

Although not many writers address peer supervision groups specifically, many suggest that it can be useful. Gold (2006), for example, says that consultation with a senior colleague in specific incidents or arranging supervision on an ongoing basis can assist clinicians in all settings and circumstances. Experienced clinicians, who may feel too advanced in their careers to put themselves in a traditional supervisory relationship but want an ongoing situation in which to present their difficult cases, may find a solution in a peer supervision group.

Supporting the concept of peer groups, Brugger, Caesar, Frank, and Marty (1962) suggest that peer group supervision made discussion of countertransference issues easier, that group members were less anxious about revealing themselves than in staff supervision, and that peers were less likely to take on a therapist role with their peers. Mintz (1968) found that experienced clinicians in a supervisory group needed very little direction from the supervisor, and tended to focus most on countertransference, both of which tend to support the idea that peer supervision is the ideal situation for experienced therapists. Counselman and Gumpert (1993) point out that the "opportunity to comment on peers' cases dilutes the regressive pull of the supervisory situation" (p. 27). Norman and Salomonsson (2005) discuss a specific method for presenting material in a psychoanalytically oriented peer group, a kind of free-floating "weaving thoughts" approach that they believe bypasses some of the pitfalls of intellectual debate.

Shatan, Brody, and Ghent (1962) suggest the use of peer group supervision while therapists are still in training as a way of helping them stay aware of countertransference issues. Winstead, Bonovitz, Gale, and Evans (1974) also recommend peer group supervision for people in training, and suggest that issues come up there that might not arise in traditional supervision.

Although Phillips and Kanter (1984) do not write specifically about peer supervision groups, their comments and conclusions are relevant. They find that mutuality, the quality of shared participation and interchange of thoughts and feelings, is a key element of the supervisory relationship in general and a specific component in contracting for supervision and in developing therapeutic skills. "The present authors would not limit the concept to any one model of supervision. Rather, they assert that for supervision to be effective, it must be a mutual experience offering both participants opportunities to learn and change" (p. 179). This points in the direction of peer supervision groups.

According to Shultz and Stoeffler (1986), supervision is still essential for experienced therapists, and they describe a "supervision retreat" in which a group of 8 senior therapists met once a year for daily peer supervision. I think we might suggest that once a year, while better than not at all, is hardly sufficient.

Although Hogan (1964) does not address peer supervision groups specifically, the idea comes up nonetheless. He discusses a cycle of four stages of professional development that may be repeated many times. He lists "(1) method of choice, promulgated by his training, (2) adaptation of this method to his own personality, (3) reversal of method-person balance wherein his approach to therapy is a reflection of his own personal idiom through one or more methods, (4) creative approaches which are an outgrowth of both method and person. At the fourth level the supervisor takes on the role of peer supervisor rather than control supervisor" (p. 139). "During the first stage, or Level 1, his approach is heavily influenced by a method, the 'method of choice' promulgated by his training. In the second stage, or Level 2, he adapts this method to his own personality, his own idiom. In the third stage, or Level 3, the method-person balance is reversed, and his approach to therapy is a reflection of his personal idiom through one or more methods. In the fourth stage, or Level 4, he goes beyond method and his own personal idiom to develop creative approaches which are an outgrowth of both method and person" (p. 139). "At this stage [level 4], I believe the *control supervisor model is far infe-*

*rior to the peer supervisor model*" (p. 141, italics mine). I think this is a strong endorsement of the peer supervision group.

Weaks (2002) identified core conditions necessary for an effective supervisory relationship to become established: equality, safety and challenge. Equality is more likely to be found in a peer relationship than in a traditional training situation. Akhurst and Kelly (2006) discuss adding peer supervision to an already-existing training program, because it allows for a "different form of learning experience" (p. 3) that complements and supplements the traditional modes of training. Todd and Pine (1968) found that a long-term peer supervision group helped minimize countertransferential reactions and helped the members continue to improve their clinical skills.

In a survey of 563 psychologists, Lewis, Greenburg, and Hatch (1988) found that 23 percent were members of a peer supervision group at the time and another 60 percent expressed the desire to join a group if there was one available. They described the structure of the typical peer group as follows: "The typical peer consultation group is formed through personal contact. Members rotate the hosting of the meetings, which are regularly scheduled in their homes and offices. The group is informal, small (6 persons), and leaderless with a spontaneous format. When members drop out, new members are added casually through sponsorship of one member and group consensus. The group's time is spent helping each member with the difficult cases presented at each meeting, discussing professional/ethical issues, and giving emotional support" (p. 85). In its generalizations, this description is close to what we found.

In one of the few articles specifically about peer supervision groups, Counselman and Weber (2004) suggest that the potential benefits are many: reducing the isolation of private practice, presenting a wide spectrum of solutions to clinical problems, preventing clinical burnout, reducing therapist shame about errors and personal limitations, and offering a forum for continuing learning and experience. They make the point that peer supervision groups are really consultation groups, rather than supervision groups, since supervision entails some differential in authority, and the supervisor often shares responsibility for the patients.

Counselman and Weber describe the "well-functioning" peer supervision group (p. 133) as sharing the tasks of leadership, which for them include "adherence to contract, gatekeeping and boundary management, and working with resistance" (p. 133). A successful peer supervision group stays with its original purpose, "does not become a therapy group or social event, although the pulls in both directions are quite strong" (p. 133), and "does not allow a de facto leader to emerge" (p. 133). Gatekeeping functions, managing the leaving of old members and joining of new ones, must also be addressed. "Flexible membership boundaries allow departing members to be replaced, thus insuring the continued life of the group" (p. 135).

Counselman and Weber mention certain dangers that may undermine the functioning of a peer supervision group. Fear of being criticized can lead to a group becoming "too nice" (p. 131), where members do not challenge each other sufficiently, so that learning and personal growth are stunted. Another danger Counselman and Weber describe is failure to sufficiently process real events in the group, such as member deaths or departures. Any conflict that occurs must also be directly addressed and not ignored. "A group needs to be in agreement on the value of talking about group process" (p. 138). Some groups are resistant to doing this kind of work. Counselman and Weber (2004) say that "there should be a clear contract, understood by all" (p.133), but I have found that most of the people interviewed were unable to articulate a contract other than the agreement about confidentiality.

Goldberg (1981) also writes specifically about peer supervision groups, and his own experiences in different groups. He finds that there is "clearly a need for practitioners to find an opportunity for exchange with trusted colleagues, for the evocation of deeply encountered feelings about their work and the processes and directions toward which they aspire as purposive beings" (p. 27). Goldberg mentions four reasons peer supervision groups are formed: clinical—peer supervision is more appropriate for experienced therapists; professional—it can become a source of referrals as one's professional competence is demonstrated; emotional—the group provides support, encouragement, and a safe place to discharge negative feelings about the work; and social—the group is an antidote to the isolation of private practice. He also investigates the areas of group functioning that he believes should be addressed in forming or joining a group: the purpose of the group; the frequency, duration, and location of meetings; adding new members; losing members; contact outside the group; the composition of the group; the personal attributes of the members, including their amount of personal therapy and existential concerns; the group process itself; commitment, attention, and attendance; development of trust and the modes of participation; overprotecting other members; handling conflict; and several other issues. Another area he mentions is the question of rotating leadership, which he seems to favor, referencing and quoting Nobler (1980), although it appears to me that it defeats the purpose of peer supervision. The group Nobler describes sounds more like a therapy group than a peer supervision group, and while it is certainly possible to have a leaderless therapy group, even one with rotating leadership, that is quite a different thing from the peer

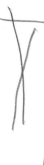

supervision group that most people want. Surprisingly, Goldberg appears to have had many negative experiences, and seems suspicious of people's motives for joining, for example, a "dysfunctional attempt to get help for serious personal problems" (p. 29), or a "greater investment in being liked than an openness for learning" (p. 29). Hardly anyone interviewed for this book indicated that there was someone like that in his or her group.

In another positive take on peer groups, Billow and Mendelsohn (1987) describe a spectrum that ranges between case-centered peer supervision groups and process-centered groups. Case-centered groups focus on the clinical material; process-centered groups focus on "the detailed investigation of the here and now of the peer group" (p. 38); dual-focus groups relate "the here-and-now of group experience to case material" (p. 45). Most groups seem to do at least a little of both. They also point out that the "very act of presentation to the peer supervisory group, and the preparation for it, may actually have powerful effects on the treatment relationship itself" (p. 42).

In a related vein, Kline (1972, 1974) describes a leaderless therapy group, which functions well because the members temporarily assume and then relinquish the role of leader, as needed. He found that all the usual experiences of transference, projection, and the other feelings that developed between the members were successfully explored, discussed, and examined in the group. His finding that this therapy group did not need a formal leader to control the group has positive implications for the concept of a peer supervision group, which also meets without a leader.

Schröder and Davis (2004) developed a system for analyzing and categorizing therapist difficulties, finding that most fell into one of three categories: *transient,* or those resulting from a competency deficit in the therapist; *paradigmatic,* or those resulting from the character and personality of the therapist; and *situational,* or those resulting from the particulars of the patient or the therapeutic situation. With experienced clinicians, the peer group is well suited to deal with all of these, but may be especially helpful in addressing the paradigmatic type, what we usually call *countertransference.*

One of the ways peer supervision may have an advantage is in the use of parallel process. McNeill and Worthen (1989) discuss the use of parallel process interventions in supervision, and conclude that "the parallel process in supervision in its various manifestations can be the focus for some of the most potent and impactful interventions within the supervisory relationship. Consequently, we suggest that supervisors pay close attention to the process in order to facilitate effective supervision, as well as personal and professional growth in psychotherapy trainees"

(p. 333). They caution that, in individual or group supervision with a supervisor, there may be ethical dilemmas, in that "the notion of addressing personal or parallel process issues may take on connotations of a supervision/therapy overlap. As a result, supervisors may be reluctant to discuss these issues in supervision for fear of placing themselves in an ethical dilemma concerning the dual role as supervisor and personal therapist for a trainee. We underscore the point that supervision should not be personal therapy and that confusing the boundaries between supervision and personal therapy for a trainee clearly results in a conflicting dual-role relationship" (p. 332). Peer group supervision eliminates this dilemma.

The Supervisory Relationship:
Individual Sup.

Group Sup:

Peer Sup:
Case Centered : Clinical material
process centered : detailed investig of the here
and now
dual focused group : Relate here and now
to the case material.

The problem of supervision:

Structure:    Contract/agrement.

Training and Competence:

Supervisors Responsivenus:

Shame:

# Chapter 2

# The Problems of Supervision

As positive an experience as it may sometimes be, we must recognize that there are some issues and difficulties with supervision as it is practiced today. The way supervisors are trained (or not trained at all), and their competence (or lack of it) in the role can lead to negative experiences for their supervisees. The very structure of the supervisory situation can infantilize or shame the trainee and lead to resentment and the concealing of information.

## Structure

There are a number of problems with the traditional format for supervision of psychotherapy. In many supervision situations, the contract about what the supervisor and the trainee are doing is never discussed. Teitelbaum (1990) says that the supervisor and the therapist-in-training have to discuss and negotiate a clear and mutually agreed-upon contract, something he suggests often does not happen, leading to misunderstandings and misalliances. He also says that supervisors may be reluctant to take responsibility for problems in the supervision, and may blame them on the inexperience or even the pathology of the supervisee. Whitman (2001, Whitman & Jacobs, 1998) emphasizes the importance of educating both supervisor and student in the structure and content of supervision. She points out that trainees may also be uneducated about how to use supervision and what the contract is with the supervisor. She found that even a one-hour session covering the contract/agreement, the characteristics of a good supervisor, and how to address a problem helped trainees feel more comfortable and more open.

Phillips and Kanter (1984) also discuss the contract. "From the outset it is critical that the supervisor and supervisee establish a well-defined contract for supervision. The supervisee is invited to detail what is desired from supervision; the supervisor also presents what is offered. A groundwork of mutuality is laid involving agreement about what is to be worked on, mutual understanding about how this is to be done and over what period of time, and articulation of expectations of supervisor and supervisee. Out of the negotiated interchange a formal working arrangement is outlined describing what will happen in supervision" (p. 180).

Nelson and Friedlander (2001) also found problems in the contract. "In a majority of the cases, there was a disagreement about what should take place in supervision. Frequently the supervisees experienced a desire for more time and input from the supervisor than they were receiving. A concern voiced by numerous participants was uncertainty about the supervisor's commitment to them or a lack of clarity about the supervision contract" (p. 390).

Part of the problem may be improved by better educating supervisees about the supervisory situation. Kennard, Stewart, and Gluck (1987) found that "[s]upervisors have better experiences with trainees who are perceived as interested in the supervisor's opinions and formulations about the trainees' development and behavior. These data raise the question of whether instructors can teach trainees to be better supervisees by learning specific behaviors" (p. 174). Kennard, Stewart, and Gluck (1987) emphasize that supervisee enthusiasm may be a significant factor for the supervisor. "When the supervisor perceives the trainee as interested in feedback and in suggestions regarding professional development, trainees report a better experience in supervision. Trainees report positive experiences with supervisors who are more supportive, instructional, and interpretive. Similarities along the dimensions of theoretical orientation and behavioral style appear to be important contributors to the match. Trainees who have positive supervision experiences perceive themselves as interpretive with their clients in therapy and likewise perceive the supervisor as interpretive in supervision. The discriminant analysis suggests a hierarchy of behavioral style contributors to positive versus negative experiences" (p. 174).

In a review of much of the research on supervision, Worthington (1987) found that, while adjusting the supervision to the level of experience of the supervisee is a nice idea in theory, in reality it happens very little. He "found that supervisors did not make differential discrimination of counselor needs as counselors gained experience" (p. 205). Yogev and Pion (1984) also found "that supervisors do not modify their way of providing supervision according to supervisees' level of experience and/or in response to the different needs supervisees have at each stage" (p. 207).

Murray (1974) found a problem in the very nature of the relationship itself. "The vast majority of students and supervisors described their relationship as a teacher–student relationship. In addition, 60 per cent of the faculty believe that the students want such a relationship. However, 92 per cent of the students claim to want an *equal* [author's italics] relationship in which one professional relates to another" (p. 293). He also found a discrepancy between students and supervisors, that while "the majority of supervisors say they are interested in the students' ideas and suggestions, a third of the students feel that their supervisor has no interest in the students' ideas and opinions" (p. 293).

Introducing a special issue on psychotherapy training, Ladany (2007) suggests that many assumptions about supervision may be questionable, even specious. "With most of the focus on knowledge, it would arguably seem, looking from the outside, that knowledge gained is the primary outcome of graduate training, with psychotherapy skills coming in a distant second, and self-awareness coming sometime after lunch. It is conceivable that the assumption that knowledge gained leads to more effective psychotherapists is, at best, a tenuous assumption" (p. 392). We know from much research that the personality and personal character of  the therapist matter much more than his or her theoretical orientation or level of training (Hubble, Duncan, & Miller, 1999). Ladany (2007) goes on to question assumptions about training in general. "In all likelihood, coursework, at best, offers a foundation of understanding about psychotherapy that may or may not actually lead to, or be directly linked to, psychotherapy competence" (p. 392). "Without personal therapy, I believe that therapists quickly hit a wall of growth that in turn limits their effectiveness as therapists" (p. 393).

Ladany (2007) puts tremendous emphasis on the importance of "helping skills." "In fact, I would argue that helping skills training is the most important training experience in graduate school. Indeed, if psychotherapy graduate programs could only offer two courses, they should both be on developing competence in helping skills. Unfortunately, helping skills have typically warranted the least amount of formal time, if any is allocated at all" (p. 394). He believes that "a relatively large percentage of therapists enter graduate school with a low ability for helping, and the difference between these students and those who do not enter graduate school may not be as stark as suggested. In addition, this same large percentage who enter graduate school with low ability leave it as mediocre to poorly functioning therapists. As a field, we have not properly considered the gatekeeping role, and as a result, we are graduating many therapists who have no business functioning in the role as therapists" (p. 394).

Questioning the selection of candidates, Ladany (2007) goes on to comment on the process of admission into the training program itself. He seems to imply that at least some of the problems inherent in supervision are due to the caliber of the trainees, suggesting that "much of the decisions made regarding admittance into a psychotherapy training programs are based on criteria that have little relation to psychotherapy competence, or, I would argue, even the potential for psychotherapy competence (i.e., grades, GRE scores, money, research experience, unreliable interviews, etc.). Once in graduate school, it is rather difficult to gatekeep or even reroute students who may be deemed poor therapists (in large part because of the variability in competence among the faculty and supervisors). It should not surprise us, then, that a decent percentage of students graduate are not well equipped to be reasonably good therapists. A good litmus test for this supposition is to ask ourselves whether we would refer a family member (that we liked!) to a therapist whom we are graduating. I would venture a guess that about a third of the time the answer would be no" (p. 395).

## Training and Competence

Another problem arising in supervision is that supervisors may not know how to supervise. It appears to be assumed that experienced clinicians will know how to be a good supervisor, but this may not always be the case. Teitelbaum (1995) suggests that "in addition to experience, a separate set of acquired skills is now necessary to become a capable supervisor" (p. 184). O'Connor (2000) says that American Psychological Association guidelines are ambiguous and contribute to creating less than optimal supervisory practices. West (2003) in Britain says that "[i]t is suggested that a professional culture of supervision has been constructed that may not reflect the best interests of either clients or practitioners" (p. 123).

Robiner and Schofield (1990) published a bibliography of publications on supervision in psychotherapy and more generally in professional psychology, especially during internship. They found that supervisors often lack training in how to supervise. "Although supervision is within the top five activities that psychologists spend the most professional time on, and more than two thirds of counseling psychologists provide clinical supervision, few supervisors (less than 10% to 15%) actually have attended formal courses in supervision, most lack training in supervision, little is known about how supervisors assume the supervisory role, the full extent of supervisors' responsibilities and legal liabilities are not necessarily evident to supervisees or supervisors, and standardized rating scales for assessing supervisees' and supervisors' skills are wanting. There is no solid theoretical base, standard literature or syllabus for supervision: assigning readings about supervision ranks seventh among supervisory techniques; fewer than 20% of supervisors frequently recommend such readings. No model training sequence in supervision has been developed or adopted by professional or accreditation organizations. Although the 'master therapist' model of supervision may be popular, there is consensus neither on who should become a supervisor, nor on when sufficient clinical, research, or supervised experience in an area invests a person with the requisite expertise to assume supervisory responsibilities. Guidelines and standards are lacking for interdisciplinary and postdoctoral supervision, as well as for ongoing supervision (as mandated in some states), of impaired psychological practitioners or those with subdoctoral training" (p. 297–298).

In an update of Robiner and Schofield (1990), Peake, Nussbaum, and Tindell (2002) address updated issues in supervision, such as the call for empirically supported treatments, brief therapy models, and changing ethics in an environment influenced by cost containment. "The American Psychological Association (1996), in revamping its guidelines for accrediting doctoral and internship programs, has included such training as a crucial part of the curriculum" (p. 114). Peake, Nussbaum, and Tindell acknowledge the importance of the relationship between the supervisor and the supervisee. "Training, skills, and quality of the relationship are the core dimensions in supervision. The student looks to his or her supervisor not just as a teacher but also as a role model—even a confidant. It is difficult to trust your fears, doubts, and questions to someone with whom you are not comfortable. The students know the supervisor will see them stumble, and it is up to them to convey the importance of honesty and scholarly discussion as a means of professional growth. Researchers have been visiting these topics much more frequently in the past decade. Deciding how supervision is best delivered is a challenging, but exciting, task" (p. 116).

Although her book is generally very positive about the enterprise of supervision, Alonso (1985) acknowledges that "it has been the tradition that once one finishes being trained as a psychotherapist, one is ready to begin supervising. Many promising supervisors are so disheartened by finding themselves pressed into service with little or no supervisory training that they flee the role and are lost forever to the profession"

(p. 6). Alonso (1985) acknowledges that the supervisor can contribute or even cause a conflict or impasse. Certain qualities in the supervisor can create these difficulties, and she lists "1) the need to be admired; 2) the need to rescue; 3) the need to be in control; 4) the need to compete; 5) the need to be loved; 6) . . . unresolved conflicts from the supervisor's own training experience; and 7) spillover from personal stress in the personal or professional life of the supervisor" (p. 88). Alonso understands that the situation can be shaming for the supervisor. "Supervisors . . . find it awkward to discuss their ignorance with colleagues and to ask for help in what is supposed to be their area of expertise" (p. 6).

Watkins (1990, 1992, 1995a,b,c, 1996, 1997) has written extensively about supervision and gives specific descriptions and recommendations for improving the process. He says that, in spite of the importance of supervision in the training of therapists, supervisors are often undertrained. Watkins (1990) says "we have no real substantive models that explicate the developmental process supervisors themselves go through in becoming supervisors, we have few studies about supervisors' acquisition of supervisory skills, and we have few studies that examine the changes resulting from supervisors' accumulation of supervisory experience" (p. 553), and offers a 4-stage model of psychotherapy supervisor development: role shock, role recovery and transition, role consolidation, and role mastery.

Also calling into question the abilities of the supervisor, Salvendy (1993) points out that, despite the importance of supervisors in the careers of fledgling group therapists, "the specific preparation of the supervisors for their task is quite unsystematic and lacking" (p. 365), and the selection of a supervisor "is still haphazard and often dictated by politics and power" (p. 365). Gill (2001), in a more recent publication, believes that supervisors today more often accept their part in supervisory conflicts and stalemates, and that they now recognize that supervision may be more difficult and arouse more anxiety than the supervisee's own therapy or analysis. Barnat (1973) found that "[i]nadequate supervision may result in the clinical trainee losing himself in partial, temporary identifications or, worse, it may preclude identification, and therefore crucial learning, altogether" (p. 17). The most common issues in the supervisor were "supervisory affectation, exclusively technical zeal, and role rigidity" (p. 22).

In a somewhat disturbing article, Allen, Szollos, and Williams (1986) found that the "[w]orst supervision experiences apparently were harder for our respondents to define by citing the presence of specific characteristics. Rather, they seemed better identifiable through the absence of effective teaching strategies and role modeling. A majority of poor supervisors were characterizable as disinterested or inept, and a minority as authoritarian or exploitative. Students in a vast majority of worst supervisory situations found themselves at the mercy of supervisors who conveyed subtle disinterest in the process (e.g., spending less time, relying more on student self-reports as opposed to observing trainees, and so forth). Authoritarian denigration was most apparent in efforts by worst supervisors to encourage conformity and to punish divergence from the 'party line.' The laissez faire and authoritarian styles of supervision are both related to lowered levels of trainee satisfaction. . . . The effects of subtle neglect inherent in laissez faire supervision are especially difficult to ferret out" (p. 98).

On a dark note, Worthington (1987) came to this very disappointing conclusion about supervisors: "Supervisors do not become more competent as they gain experience" (p. 203).

## Supervisor Responsiveness

Gray, Ladany, Walker, and Ancis (2001) did a study that identified many different kinds of negative interactions with supervisors, which ruptured the relationship in the same ways as would happen to a therapist with a patient. They found that "a plausible explanation for nondisclosure is that the trainees did not perceive their supervisors to be receptive to hearing their disclosures of counterproductive supervision experiences" (p. 380). Trainees did not always blame the supervisor. "An interesting finding that emerged from the data is that trainees found ways to justify the counterproductive event. Many trainees attributed partial blame for the counterproductive event to themselves, and several defended their supervisors. According to cognitive dissonance theory, perhaps the presence of trainee self-blame relates to the severity of counterproductive events. For example, the more damaging the counterproductive event, the more trainees may seek to justify the event's occurrence to ease the cognitive dissonance caused by a respected authority behaving in a harmful way" (p. 380). They also found that "trainees typically did not disclose their experience of a counterproductive event to their supervisors. Most attributed their nondisclosure to a poor supervisory relationship. In just fewer than half of the cases, trainees and supervisors discussed the counterproductive event. Of these disclosures, only one supervisor initiated the discussion" (p. 380).

Similarly, Murray (1974) found that "[m]any student responses indicate that problems may be due to lack of supervisor commitment. Supervisors corroborate this, as one out of four faculty members stated that they did not spend sufficient time carrying out supervisory duties or that supervision was the lowest priority among their professional duties. The entire faculty saw themselves as standing up for the students without reservations in time of trouble, but 36% of the students felt they could count on their supervisor's support only if his position was not in jeopardy" (p. 293). This is another issue that may be avoided in a peer group.

In another study, Moskowitz and Rupert (1983) interviewed 158 graduate students in clinical psychology about conflicts in their supervisory experiences. Over a third (38 percent) reported a major conflict with a supervisor that made it difficult to learn from supervision. These conflicts occurred in three major areas: theoretical orientation or therapeutic approach, style of supervision, and personality issues. Some kinds of conflicts, i.e., conflicts that centered on style of supervision were easier to resolve than personality issues. When conflicts were unresolved, trainees looked for support from others, stopped revealing difficulties to the supervisor, or appeared to comply with the supervisor.

Nelson and Friedlander (2001) did a revealing study in which thirteen master's level and doctoral trainees were interviewed about a supervision experience that had a detrimental effect on their training. They point out that this area, while important, is rarely examined. "Little is known, however, about how trainees actually cope with highly conflicted supervisory relationships" (p. 384). They were surprised by their findings. "Whereas the authors expected to hear tales of important lessons imparted by supervisors, most informants described a lack of investment on the part of the supervisors, little support for trainee autonomy, and an absence of confirmation for the supervisees' strengths" (p. 385). Nelson and Friedlander (2001) found that the quality of the supervisory relationship was crucial. "Two major patterns emerged in participants' descriptions of how they experienced the establishment of their supervisory relationships. The most typical pattern involved supervisors who were viewed as remote and uncommitted to establishing a strong training relationship. Perceiving their supervisors as too busy to bother with their training needs, the supervisees felt uncomfortable or disappointed with their supervisors from the beginning" (p. 387). Nelson and Friedlander (2001) also found that the question of who is the senior clinician, and who is in charge, can arise. "The most pervasive, although not universal, pattern in this study was the occurrence of a power struggle or role conflict between supervisor and supervisee. This condition was often observed in dyads in which the supervisee seemed to have greater status than the supervisor in some way. Frequently, the supervisee reportedly had considerable clinical experience before entering the supervision relationship. In some cases, the supervisee seemed to have had expertise in one or more areas that the supervisor did not, or the supervisee was older and had more life experience than the supervisor. In most of these cases, the trainees felt that the supervisors reacted as if threatened" (p. 389).

Surprisingly, supervisors can react in ways that verge on abusive. "According to respondents, the predominant supervisor reaction to the conflicts was ongoing, extensive anger. Supervisees frequently described feeling scapegoated by their supervisors, and a variant number were criticized openly in front of peers or other colleagues" (Nelson and Friedlander, 2001, p. 390). Even when not actively abusive, supervisors can lose the trust of their supervisees. "Typically, supervisees experienced lack of support from their supervisors. Most lost trust in their supervisors, felt unsafe, pulled back from the relationship, and maintained a guarded stance in supervision. Typically, supervisees experienced a sense of powerlessness. This was expressed frequently in terms of feeling manipulated or in terms of a violation of boundaries. A minority believed that their life experiences, skills, or differences were not valued by the supervisor, and others felt 'written off'" (p. 390–391). Similarly, "[m]ost of the supervisees in this study did not experience enough attention, warmth, or understanding to maintain a sense of trust in their supervisors" (p. 392). Supervisors can misuse the power of their role. "Frequently, our participants described their supervisors as responding to challenges by pulling rank in an authoritarian fashion, rather than attempting to make emotional connections and build from there" (p. 392). Trainees in Australia had similar types of negative experiences (Kozlowska, Nunn, & Cousens, 1997a, b).

According to Nelson and Friedlander (2001), negative behavior on the part of the supervisor can damage the trainee. "Most, but not all, of the participants indicated that they had experienced moderate to extreme self-doubt as a result of their interactions with their supervisors" (p. 391). "Many of the participants we interviewed described being deeply hurt and confused by their experiences in supervision" (p. 391). "Despite the fact that most of our participants indicated having gained in self-awareness and confidence as a result of the experiences they recounted, these experiences nonetheless exacted a toll on their health and well-being and their sense of trust in others, particularly in authority figures. Although we have no information about how the experiences they described affected participants as counselors, it is reasonable to assume that harmful conflict in supervision detracts from a trainee's efficacy with clients. Consideration for clients, trainees, and supervisors, taken together with the painful events we heard in the course of this study, underscores a need for safeguards for both counseling and supervising students in training. Supervisor training in conflict resolution strategies may provide more support for supervisors who face inevitable interpersonal challenges with their trainees" (p. 394).

On a more positive note, Nelson and Friedlander (2001) offer some suggestions for the repair of the situation. "First, the problems need to be openly addressed and defined. If problems are a result of misunderstanding about the goals and tasks of the supervisee's training experience, clarification of the supervisee's roles and responsibilities may resolve the impasse. If the problems are more related to misunderstanding in the supervisory relationship itself, then an examination of the dynamics of the interaction may be necessary. Like psychotherapy, supervision has the potential to provide a corrective emotional experience for the supervisee when the supervisor displays openness to the supervisee's discomfort, insight about the conflict, and willingness to adapt. The supervisee who directly experiences productive conflict resolution with a supervisor will be better equipped to provide such experiences for clients" (p. 393).

A significant finding Nelson (1978) emphasized was "that the trainees valued interest in supervision over all other supervisor characteristics, including experience as a therapist and theoretical or technical knowledge. This finding suggests, on the one hand, that strong interest on the part of a supervisor may compensate somewhat for limited expertise and result in a positive learning experience for the trainee. On the other hand, extensive experience and knowledge, however valuable for the supervisor's professional functioning, may be of limited value to the trainee if substantial interest in providing supervision is absent" (p. 548).

# Shame

Shame and self-criticism can interfere with trainees presenting material to a supervisor. Talbot (1995) advises exploring this shame directly, and suggests that doing so may improve both the supervision and the therapy. Wallace and Alonso (1994) point out that adequate disclosure is essential to supervision, because the supervisor depends on information provided by the trainee to broaden and deepen understanding of the patient and to foster development of the trainee's psychotherapeutic skills. But the supervisee must feel safe enough to disclose this material, and this is not always the case.

Alonso and Rutan (1988) examine the various definitions of shame and address the ways in which it is evoked in the supervisory situation. "For many reasons, the supervisory hour is the primary arena wherein the trainees' shame and guilt is both inflicted and potentially healed. Shame in supervision is generated from four major contributing factors: 1) the learning regression, 2) the patient population, 3) the supervisor's management of the supervisory hour, and 4) transference and countertransference in supervision" (pp. 576–577).

The evocation of shame may be intrinsic to the supervisory relationship. "The learning regression is stimulated by the very nature of the supervisory process. Trainees are asked to expose their work and to put themselves on the line to their supervisors at a time when their healthy narcissistic equilibrium is under considerable stress" (p. 577). "In addition, they are usually worried about what harm they may do to their patients—and what retaliatory harm may be inflicted on them by the supervisors and administrators of their professional training" (Alonso & Rutan, p. 577).

Some of the problem comes from the supervisor. "A great deal of shame and guilt in supervision flows from the supervisor's confused and sometimes faulty notion of whether to behave like a mentor, a teacher, or a therapist to the trainee. The supervisor needs to somehow balance the didactic needs of the trainees and their very real need for concrete support with an effort to model somewhat for them how to behave with their patients. This is an inherent conflict in the supervisory role" (Alonso & Rutan, pp. 578–579). This is aspect of supervision that is mitigated by a peer supervision group, where the role of each member may be clearer.

Yourman (2003, Yourman & Farber, 1996) also found that trainees consciously conceal and distort in presentation of cases to supervisors, and that shame is often a factor in these instances. "By its very nature, psychotherapy supervision is an endeavor in which trainees are likely to experience feelings of self-doubt and shame. Because shame is an affect that often provokes a desire to hide oneself, it follows that supervisees experiencing more shame will be less likely to be forthcoming, especially about material that might be viewed negatively by their supervisors. The material most often withheld by trainees pertains to problems within the supervisory relationship. It appears that trainee shame and nondisclosure have the greatest impact upon the quality of the psychotherapy supervision itself, as opposed to the treatment being supervised" (2003, p. 601).

## Withholding Information

In most fields the trainee is watched directly in real time. A surgeon in training does surgery with his teacher at his side commenting and correcting as he goes. Because of the private and confidential nature of psychotherapy, this is not normally possible (an exception is the room with a one-way mirror and phone). It might be hard to imagine the surgeon-in-training describing a recent surgery to his supervisor as an acceptable way of learning. Yet this is how most psychotherapists get their training. The supervisor depends on the disclosures of the trainee. But what happens when crucial information is withheld?

Ladany, Hill, Corbett, and Nutt (1996) found in a study that trainees were likely to withhold information in supervision. The type of information most likely to be withheld was a negative reaction to the supervisor. Some material feels too personal to disclose, especially in institutional settings where consequences may be expected. Interestingly and importantly for this book, these nondisclosures to the supervisor were often discussed with a peer. Yourman and Farber (1996) found that while "most of the time supervisees communicate to their supervisors what they believe to be an honest picture of their interactions with their psychotherapy patients" (p. 570), almost forty percent of the time they failed to inform the supervisor about a clinical error. They also found that when the trainee disagreed with the supervisor they often concealed their disagreement. "Similarly, for the item 'When I have thought that my supervisor was wrong I have let him/her know it,' 30.1% of the sample indicated that they never or only infrequently . . . disclosed such thoughts to their supervisor. And 47.3% of the sample reported telling their supervisor what he/she wanted to hear at a moderate to high frequency. . . . In addition, 59.1% of the sample reported that they never or only infrequently felt comfortable disclosing negative feelings toward their supervisor" (p. 571). The more unsatisfied the trainee was with the supervisor, the more often that dissatisfaction was concealed. "Two items, supervisee satisfaction and discussion of countertransference, were found to be significantly related to nondisclosure/distortion; the higher the frequency score on these items, the less trainee nondisclosure/distortion was reported" (p. 571).

In their survey, Ladany and colleagues (1996) found that "most supervisees (97.2%) do withhold information from their supervisors. The content of the nondisclosures most often involved negative reactions to the supervisor, personal issues not directly related to supervision, clinical mistakes, evaluation concerns, general client observations, and, to a lesser extent, negative reactions to clients, countertransference, client-counselor attraction issues, positive reactions to the supervisor, supervision setting concerns, supervisor appearance, supervisee-supervisor attraction issues, and positive reactions to clients. The most typical reasons for the nondisclosures were perceived unimportance, the personal nature of the nondisclosure, negative feelings about the nondisclosure, a poor alliance with the supervisor, deference to the supervisor, impression management, and, to a lesser extent, the supervisor's agenda, political suicide, pointlessness, and a belief that the supervisor was not competent" (pp. 17–18).

When a supervisee concealed something from the supervisor, they often found other people to help process the problem. Ladany and colleagues (1996) found "that most (66%) of the nondisclosures were discussed with someone other than the supervisor. Thus, supervisees frequently availed themselves of other sources with whom to disclose. The most typical person to whom supervisees turned was a peer or friend in the field (53%)" (p. 15). When they are dissatisfied with the supervisor, trainees often create a peer supervision setting on their own.

Ladany, Friedlander, and Nelson (2005b) examined pivotal experiences in supervision. They found certain difficulties inherent in the supervisory situation. "When asked to disclose personal information, the supervisee may feel defensive or threatened, believing that the supervisor sees personal or professional inadequacy" (p. 80). "Other markers of role conflict include the supervisee's (a) direct or indirect (sarcasm, defensiveness) expression of anger or other negative feelings about the supervisor or supervisory process; (b) expressed disagreement about the goals or tasks of supervision or about the supervisor's evaluation; (c) overcompliance (rapid agreement with the supervisor without exploration or elaboration, i.e., 'lip service'); (d) noncompliance (nonresponsiveness or begrudging acceptance of the supervisor's input); (e) avoidance (arriving late, canceling, or failing to attend supervision, coming unprepared, ignoring the supervisor's comments, or skipping from topic to topic); and (f) self-esteem-enhancing behaviors, such as justification or self-aggrandizing" (p. 84).

Normalizing the situation, Yerushalmi (1992) suggests that there are some intrinsic characteristics of the supervisory situation that make it likely that supervisees will conceal some aspects of the clinical case being presented; that it is, in this way, natural and expectable; and that there are different types of concealment, reflecting different personality issues of the supervisee. The supervisor who understands and accepts this can use the information to better understand the supervisee. Peer supervision groups may be the antidote to many, if not all, of these problems.

Peer supervision groups are not without their problems. For example, Counselman and Gumpert (1993) suggest that leader-led groups may be more effective than peer groups because "the structural needs are managed . . . and thus can feel safer than leaderless groups" (p. 30). In another example, Hunt and Issacharoff (1975; Issacharoff & Hunt, 1977) describe a group of eleven psychiatrists and psychologists who met for three years, initially as a peer supervision group, but then they tried to turn the group into a leaderless therapy group. They suggest that a leader may be important in the functioning of a group that meets for personal growth, and that, because the members were taking the leadership role, they were unable to participate in other group processes. Nestler (1990) describes the (hopefully) unusual situation of multiple supervisors giving contradictory feedback. He seems to believe that this happens more than my own experience would suggest. However, it is one of the dangers of peer supervision, that group members may disagree about how to handle a case and not reach a consensus that the presenter can adopt.

The peer supervision group is not a perfect structure. Nevertheless, I believe that it can bypass many of the problems of the supervisory situation and provide a career-long environment of learning, safety, and support.

# Part II

# The Interviews

# Chapter 3

# Who Are the Interviewees?

No one knows how many mental health professionals in this country belong to a peer supervision group, and no one knows how many peer supervision groups there are. My best guess is that about half of the clinicians I know belong to a peer group, and half don't. My impression is that many of those who don't are still in agency positions, and have a part-time private practice. The staff meetings at the agency may meet their needs for support, connection, and collegiality. But I think they are unlikely to bring up their private patients in that setting.

In planning this book, I thought about how to most effectively describe and convey the experience of being in a peer supervision group. As in several of my other books, I decided that the best way would be to talk to the people who are actually doing it. I began with those people I knew personally and professionally, and they sometimes passed me along to other members of their group. At several professional conventions and meetings, I asked anyone in the workshops I was attending if they were a member of a peer group and if they would be willing to talk about their experience. Of those who were in a group, most (I would estimate 75 percent) agreed to participate. Those who did not agree usually said they were too busy.

This sample of peer supervision group members who agreed to be interviewed came primarily from the New York area, although several people from other parts of the country were also included. I don't believe there is any reason for regional differences in the way peer groups work, so I am reasonably sure that the responses will reflect peer groups everywhere. I don't make any claim of statistical validity for this sample, but

I do believe that they are representative of peer groups in general throughout the country. Of course, if anyone who reads this book has a very different experience I would love to hear about it.

Whenever possible, people were interviewed in person. Those individuals who live in other parts of the country, or whose schedules made it too difficult to meet in person, were interviewed by phone. In both situations, interviews were recorded and later transcribed by me. Some authors hire people to do the transcriptions, but I have found that transcribers who are not trained in psychotherapy often mishear what interviewees actually say and/or misinterpret what they mean. In addition, transcribing the recordings is a good way to familiarize myself with the material I have collected. I have lightly edited the tapes for readability and sense.

The questionnaire itself (see Appendix A) was designed over several months. I tried to cover all aspects of group functioning and of member experience. My own history in three different peer groups over the past thirty years helped me know what questions to ask. The final question (Is there anything else about your experience that we haven't covered that you want to mention?) was included in case I did overlook something, but only a few people added anything more, and that was only in the first few interviews. These topics were then added to the questionnaire.

The time the interviews took ranged from 20 minutes to 45 minutes. Most people seemed very candid and open with me. In many cases, their remarks were much longer than space allows for here. My impression in most instances was that they were clearly trying very hard to be as honest and real as they could be.

Among those interviewed, there were many different backgrounds and degrees: eighteen M.S.W. social workers, seven Ph.D. psychologists, three Ed.D. psychologists, one Psy.D. psychologist, three L.P. licensed psychoanalysts, one M.D. psychiatrist, and one N.P. nurse practitioner. This is a seasoned group with many years of clinical experience. People ranged in years of practice from six years to forty-five years of practice, with a mean of 28.8 years. Their years of experience in the peer group ranged from six months to thirty-two years, with a mean of 12.6 years. To make individuals less identifiable people's years of experience have been rounded off in multiples of five years.

A total of seventy-eight theoretical orientations and ways of thinking about a patient were identified (many people cited several): psychodynamic/psychoanalytic, twenty-one; eclectic, fourteen; interpersonal and/or relational, nine; cognitive/behavioral, eight; systemic/family systems, five; object relations, five; ego psychology, four; self psychology, three; trauma, three; modern analytic, two; solution-focused, imago, gestalt, and dialectical behavior therapy (DBT), one each.

There were thirty-four interviews in total. This is a completely arbitrary number. I could have done more interviews, but stopped because I was getting a lot of repetition, similar responses, and not much that was new. There were twenty-four women and ten men, from twenty different groups. I don't think this means that women are more likely to be in a peer supervision group, but it might mean exactly that. Perhaps men are more cautious about revealing how they work, and thus declined to participate.

As I discuss in Part I, the section on supervision, there is for many professionals an undercurrent of shame about revealing their work. This may contribute to therapists avoiding peer group membership, and may even underlie their believing their own rationalizations about being too busy or finding it impossible to find a group. It might also explain the refusal of those peer group members who declined to be interviewed.

I believe that the professionals who did agree to be interviewed are typical and representative of our field, and that their experiences are also typical and representative of those in peer groups everywhere.

*Shame about revealing their work !*

# Chapter 4

# The Members of the Group

Whether there are three people or twelve, somehow professionals find a way to come together and establish themselves as a group. Some groups contain new practitioners who join together after completing their training. Other groups consist of seasoned professionals who know they need feedback and help. In this chapter we will look at how people find a group, or form a group. We learn why people wanted to be in a group, and how the men and women in the group might be different.

While there are few surprises in this section, I think we get a clear sense of why peer supervision groups exist, and why people want to belong to one. We also get some simple ways to begin to participate in a group.

## How did you join the peer group?

People are either invited to join an existing group, or join with other people they know to start a new group. The interviewees were evenly divided (seventeen each) between those who had joined an existing group and those who had formed a new one. Here is a typical beginning of a new group.

A colleague in my town and I had been talking about trying to do
something professional together, because we liked each other, and he
knew another person and we knew a fourth person in common, so we
decided to start meeting. Then I brought in the fifth person.

[Female, 40 years practice, 15 years in PSG]

## Sometimes groups are very carefully crafted.

I set up the group. It's focused on sexual addiction treatment. I started
with people I knew and had supervised some of them. I wanted a group
where I really liked everyone. I also wanted people who were very
knowledgeable in sex addiction treatment. I wanted it to be diversified
in orientation and location, so I chose people who were all certified.
We did include one person who was not certified but very knowledgeable.

[Female, 30 years practice, 8 months in PSG]

Another colleague and I had been in the other group for fifteen years,
and that disbanded, and we wanted to continue to talk and explore issues pertaining to our therapy groups, so we sat down and tried to gen-
erate a list of colleagues who did group who we respected and who we
felt were capable of not just discussing cases from an intellectual perspective, but also had the capacity and openness to exploring things on a
deeper level, including any dynamics that emerged in the group itself.

[Female, 33 years practice, 2 years in PSG]

## Sometimes groups begin more spontaneously.

I went to a party and a couple of my colleagues and I were talking
about how it would be a good idea to get together and have a place
where we can talk.

[Male, 45 years practice, 20 years in PSG]

I had the idea, and got talking with a colleague who I know is interested
in marketing herself, making herself visible to the professional community around here, and I'm someone who tends to be more shy, but I
know there's value in making ourselves more visible. So we got talking
about the intersection of clinical work with the business that we're trying to maintain. So we met for coffee and found ourselves talking for
two or two and a half hours, and then we said we'd do it again. And
along the way we thought it might be fun to bring in someone else.

[Male, 12 years practice, 6 months in PSG]

When I moved from Connecticut to New York, trying to get another
practice started, I joined a kind of group practice. It was a strange insti-
tution, and I didn't stay in it very long because there was nothing about

it that agreed with my phenomenology. There were two people who I had the most significant relationships with. We started the group about six months before we left the agency, and when I left we just continued meeting.

[Female, 20 years practice, 15 years in PSG]

One of my friends said she needed a group, so we brought in some friends. We told them we wanted a place to discuss cases and get some feedback, and those first few meetings we talked about doing that, as well as doing some readings, with occasionally inviting someone in who we might have paid, consultants on different subjects.

[Female, 35 years practice, 30 years in PSG]

I set it up with my colleague. It more or less organically developed. She and I were together in the old group, and then when we moved to a bigger space we rented an extra office to a friend, and she became an automatic member. Then my colleague had another friend and he was happy to join, and then we wanted it to be a little bigger, so I invited two more people.

[Female, 25 years practice, 15 years in PSG]

## The new group may be an extension of an ongoing situation.

It was with colleagues that I did my training with. We decided to form a group.

[Female, 5 years practice, 1 year in PSG]

It was formed in the outpatient clinic. We had volunteered to get training in a specific kind of therapy, and part of that training is that we would be working together as a consultation group, and we formed that group about six months before we started the training.

[Female, 30 years practice, 3 years in PSG]

I'm one of the original members. It was through our professional organization. We all belong and there was some kind of announcement in the newsletter.

[Female, 25 years practice, 20 years in PSG]

## Very often, people are simply invited into an existing group, or ask to join a group they know is already meeting.

I was in a lunch group with some professional colleagues that meets every week, not for supervision but just for collegial support. Three of them were in a peer group already, and when mine fell apart I approached them and asked if I could join. They welcomed me.

[Female, 20 years practice, 7 years in PSG]

I had an ongoing collegial relationship with the other psychiatrist in the group, and she knew about the transition I was making in my career of doing more clinical practice, and we talked about how it would be a positive thing for me.

[Male, 40 years practice, 15 years in PSG]

**My own experience**
I have both started a group and joined existing ones, although the group I started did not last a year (see *Have you been in other peer groups?* below), and I have been in the group I joined for more than twenty-five years. Although in founding the group I was able to have a lot more control over the selection of the members, I found it a lot easier to join a group already established and coherent for several years.

# Did you know the people in the group before you joined?

Everyone knew at least one other person in the group: the person who invited them into the group. In some situations they knew everyone, because they had been together previously.

We started this group. This group came out of a reading group with a leader. We were in that group about twenty years and a group of us got very close as we got to know each other, and we began meeting and talking about cases. And we just stayed together. It was a very congenial and trusting group.

[Female, 35 years practice, 15 years in PSG]

Some people were founders of the group, and knew everyone.

They're all people I invited into the group

[Male, 40 years practice, 7 years in PSG]

Often people knew several of the members.

I always knew one person, and I met another through a weekend workshop I went to, and then I met a third, and all three were in the same group, so it seemed likely that I would try to join.

[Female, 20 years practice, 12 years in PSG]

Some people found it more difficult to join a group that had already been together for some time.

I knew them all quite well. But it's hard to go into an existing group. There's a sense of being an outsider, and of relationships already being established. That feeling has never entirely worn off.

[Female, 20 years practice, 7 years in PSG]

### My own experience

When I joined the group I am in now, I knew well only the one person who invited me into the group. I had met a few of the others at parties and other social occasions. I happened to join the group at the same time as another person I knew because she had an office in my building and we knew people in common. (She left the group after a few months.) But not being the only new person probably made it easier for me, since there was less focus exclusively on me.

I think I might have felt safe more quickly if I had known everyone, but I liked that there were people I did not know. They brought something new to me, other theoretical points of view and experiences.

## Have you been in other peer groups?

Fifteen people said they had never been in another peer supervision group. Nineteen people said they had been in other peer groups prior to the one they were in now. People left these other groups, for different reasons.

I joined an ongoing group and I think they were already having some problems. Someone had dropped out, a very divisive figure. I was with them for about a year and they decided to disband. I was disappointed because I was just getting to know them all. They assured me it had nothing to do with me. I never found out what the issues were. They said they had gotten what they were going to get from each other.

[Female, 25 years practice, 11 years in PSG]

I was in one previously for just a few years. We moved and it disbanded simultaneously. There were only four people. It was never discussed but it wasn't always helpful. There was nothing wrong with it, it just wasn't compelling.

[Female, 25 years practice, 15 years in PSG]

I was in one for about ten years that broke up because there were only three people and one got very sick and later died.

[Female, 20 years practice, 7 years in PSG]

I tried to set up another peer group around the issue of mind-body medicine, and I don't think we had a single meeting where everyone was present. Someone always had a patient emergency, or a personal crisis, or something, and the group folded after a couple of months. Either you're in it or you're not.

[Female, 40 years practice, 15 years in PSG]

Prior to this group I was in one with a group of social and community psychiatrists organized around career and administrative issues.

[Male, 40 years practice, 15 years in PSG]

For about two months, I was in a group of four or five women, and it really didn't work. We didn't bond and we didn't really get into things, discussions. I was very happy when it ended, because it wasn't working. There wasn't a good mix of personalities.

[Female, 30 years practice, 30 years in PSG]

I was, very briefly, in another group, because it just didn't work. It was a group of people I had trained with, plus a couple of add-ons, colleagues of some members. The orientations were so dissimilar that when it came to the feedback, it just didn't seem to apply. And I think the other people felt the same way. It was a kind of no-fault divorce when it ended. It's fine to have dissimilarity, but it was too divergent.

[Female, 25 years practice, 15 years in PSG]

The first lasted about six months, and the second about a year. I left the second group after being hostilely confronted by one of the other members about my verbal style and participation.

[Male, 30 years practice, 25 years in PSG]

Four of the people who said they had been in other peer supervision groups were currently in a second group, where they discussed other kinds of issues than in the group the interview focused on.

I'm in another peer group where we just deal with couples issues.

[Female, 25 years practice, 20 years in PSG]

I've also been in a family therapy peer supervision group for about twelve or fifteen years.

[Female, 35 years practice, 15 years in PSG]

I'm in a second group, something I joined about ten years ago. There are now three people in it, and we talk mostly about adult patients.

[Female, 20 years practice, 15 years in PSG]

## My own experience

I was in two other peer groups before the one I am in now, and neither of those felt right. I first sought out a peer supervision group while I was still in training. Although I had an agency position, I still wanted the holding environment of a peer group to discuss my private patients. Three of my fellow students and I formed a new group, and met for about six months. None of us knew much about group functioning, and there were probably too many issues that went unaddressed. Attendance was erratic, and two people backed out.

Eventually, the remaining two of us merged with three other people in another existing group. That worked for about a year, until I was confronted angrily about my style of participation by another member. The rest of the group was silent. We tried to address the different styles but it didn't seem to help, and I left the group feeling very hurt and misunderstood.

# What made you want to be in a peer supervision group?

People have mostly similar motivations for joining or creating a peer supervision group. Everyone has had the experience of being in supervision, and this is very often in a group. Everyone has felt the need to discuss a difficult case with a colleague.

> After we left the reading group we'd be walking around, and started talking about some of our cases. We were all very experienced, and didn't feel like we needed a supervisor, but that we could all be each other's supervisors. We wanted a place to talk about some difficulties with cases that we all had.
> [Female, 35 years practice, 15 years in PSG]

> I was trained via group supervision, and I really appreciated getting the systemic viewpoint of being in a group. When we graduated, we decided that we wanted to continue getting supervision and getting the peer support around our cases and being in private practice
> [Female, 5 years practice, 1 year in PSG]

> I was still working part-time at the hospital, where you really couldn't get that kind of peer supervision, because the focus was on administrative issues, and procedural issues. I was one of the people actually training people to do psychotherapy and crisis intervention. But there weren't very many people there who were peers, and I wanted to be with people who were respected in the field. The couple of times I at-

tended the group I was very impressed with how open they were, how supportive they were with each other, how smart they were, and I really looked forward to being able to come regularly.

[Female, 40 years practice, 17 years in PSG]

It's easy to see why people want a place to do this. In many ways, it's more difficult to understand why people wouldn't want such a group. But sometimes people aren't sure that they want a peer supervision group.

I wasn't so sure I wanted to be in such a group, but I wanted to give it a chance. On one side of the argument was that it might be good to be in a group, because this is very isolating work to do, and it would give me contact with colleagues. On the other side I was brand new, I was very unsure of myself, I didn't know if I could present a case well, or how I would be received, whether we would do a lot of literature—I didn't want to read literature. That was the ambivalence.

[Female, 30 years practice, 30 years in PSG]

Many people mentioned the isolation of private practice as a factor in wanting a peer supervision group.

Part of it was to feel a connection with the local practitioners. At that time I was working out of my house, so I was feeling very isolated, and it was really nice to get out every two weeks and discuss cases. I didn't feel like buying supervision from a senior person.

[Female, 40 years practice, 15 years in PSG]

Private practice can be pretty isolating. I had been in individual super-vision, and would be throughout my time in the group occasionally again, but I felt the need to talk to people. I had informal peer supervi-sion with colleagues when certain issues come up that I know someone is an expert on. But I wanted something more regular and structured.

[Female, 20 years practice, 12 years in PSG]

It's very lonely in private practice, and you really need other people.

[Female, 40 years practice, 18 years in PSG]

Some people mentioned the difficulty of this kind of work, especially when just starting out, and the need for support from people who under-stand.

We're working with very sick borderline patients who are highly suicidal. So the theoretical reason for being in a group is that no one person could treat these patients alone, no one could carry and contain all
that alone.

[Female, 30 years practice, 3 years in PSG]

When you're new at doing therapy, you want support, you want people
to help you when you have difficult cases, someplace that's secure in
terms of confidentiality where you talk about cases and get support.

[Female, 30 years practice, 30 years in PSG]

Many people wanted a regularly scheduled meeting where they could
bring problems and difficulties to experienced colleagues for help, sometimes with a very specific focus.

I was attracted to the idea of having a place where I could talk about
complicated clinical situations.

[Male, 40 years practice, 15 years in PSG]

I wanted for myself a place where I could talk about issues and about
cases and be with people who understood this particular type of treatment.

[Female, 30 years practice, 8 months in PSG]

This is the first group that's exclusively focused on practice development. It's not hard to find people to talk to about clinical issues, but it's
less easy to find people with whom you can talk about the hidden side
of practice, the business part, where you can talk freely about your
questions about money, about how you handle the early stages of con-
necting with a client, whether it's by phone or by email or some other
way. And talk about how we want to represent ourselves and how we
want to set up the foundation for our business.

[Male, 10 years practice, 6 months in PSG]

Many people also mentioned the desire for intellectual stimulation and
exchange of ideas and experiences.

Each of my colleagues has a different frame of reference and they're all
so bright, and I wanted the benefit of the different perspectives.

[Female, 10 years practice, 6 years in PSG]

I really benefit from talking out loud about cases, and from hearing and
listening—I don't even have to say anything—to other people talk
about their cases. It's a good learning environment for me.

[Female, 35 years practice, 2 years in PSG]

Even though I was in private supervision, I wanted to be with other therapists, see what other people were doing.

[Female, 35 years practice, 30 years in PSG]

Some others mentioned a desire for a place to learn more about themselves, and give themselves the challenge of revealing their work.

I wanted a place where I could explore myself.

[Male, 45 years practice, 5 years in PSG]

I responded to the invitation because I was aware that I hadn't had the
experience and I was aware that I haven't exposed my work recently in
that kind of an ongoing way.

[Male, 15 years practice, 1 year in PSG]

The best kind of supervision has to do with looking at yourself. This
group is in many ways a form of therapy. E. Mark Stern said it
shouldn't be called "supervision," it should be called "intervision," because we are all equals together.

[Male, 40 years practice, 7 years in PSG]

But why not paid supervision with an expert leader?

I didn't want to go to a private supervisor. I wanted to get out of the
student role.

[Female, 25 years practice, 15 years in PSG]

I wanted to learn from equals and peers. I didn't want to pay someone
anymore.

[Male, 15 years practice, 5 years in PSG]

## My own experience
Even in the middle of my training, I knew that I was going to want to be
in a peer group. Private practice seemed very isolated to me, and I
wanted to have the ongoing support of a network of people I trusted.
Even though the first group I was in had its issues and did not survive
long, the opportunity to bring in and discuss a difficult clinical problem
was extremely important and valuable.

My experiences in supervision during my training made me quite
sure that I wanted a peer supervision situation. I was very unhappy with
the power differential between supervisor and supervisee. I didn't want
to stop learning and growing as a clinician, but I was unwilling to put
myself back in the student role. I wanted to feel like a grownup, a professional who was responsible for my work and my patients, not believing

that I knew all the answers but being resourceful enough to get help finding them. Peer group provided the perfect solution.

## What is the makeup of the group?

There were thirty-four people interviewed from twenty different groups. (In some instances I interviewed more than one person from the same group.) Group size ranged from three to twelve members, with a mean of 6.26. One group of twelve was all men; two groups (of four and seven) were all women, but most groups were of mixed gender.

Some people had been in training together and had formed a group after training ended. They shared a theoretical orientation, which helped them feel understood and safe.

> We were all trained together so we had pretty much the same orientation.
>
> [Female, 5 years practice, 1 year in PSG]

In many groups there was a variety of backgrounds; this can add to the richness of the discussion.

> There are two psychologists, two psychiatrists, and two social workers. Often the two physicians will have a perspective that the rest of the group doesn't share.
>
> [Male, 40 years practice, 15 years in PSG]

> There are all different orientations, different specialties, different credentials. And the different points of view are really helpful—something I would never have thought of myself.
>
> [Female, 25 years practice, 15 years in PSG]

> We all have a similar theoretical orientation. Except one person, she has a very different point of view, but she's gotten more similar over the years. She was trained in a cognitive/behavioral orientation, but she was open to a more analytic style of thinking—that's why she joined us. Sometimes her perspective was very helpful with these very difficult cases.
>
> [Female, 20 years practice, 15 years in PSG]

> We have different orientations, which is very helpful because we can see the case from different viewpoints.
>
> [Female, 30 years practice, 30 years in PSG]

**My own experience**

Most of my professional life I have been in a large group and I like hearing a lot of different points of view. My group now has nine people, two men and seven women. Most people have a social work degree; three have a degree in psychology. The different backgrounds get expressed in different takes on a case.

# Has there been much turnover?

Most groups have some turnover; people leave for various reasons. Sometimes the spaces are filled, sometimes not.

> Some moved away, one person gave up her practice to do something else.
>
> [Female, 35 years practice, 32 years in PSG]

> One person left after a short time and it wasn't really clear why, but it was good that she left. It wasn't working for her. She didn't fit. Another person left after a pretty long time and she did fit, but she was taking on the directorship of a training program and didn't have time anymore.
>
> [Female, 25 years practice, 15 years in PSG]

Sometimes members leave the group because they are angry, unhappy, or don't fit well with the others.

> One woman left the group. It was a combination of time conflicts, but I think this person was not entirely comfortable with the level of openness, or how we were doing the group.
>
> [Female, 25 years practice, 1 year in PSG]

> One person left because they didn't fit; they didn't like us.
>
> [Female, 35 years practice, 30 years in PSG]
> Some people have left and they gave other reasons but I thought they felt that they weren't being supported; they weren't getting what they wanted.
>
> [Female, 45 years practice, 30 years in PSG]

Several groups had experienced a loss due to death of a member.

> A couple of people died untimely, one in his fifties, and one in her early sixties. Some people had left. The deaths of two people in a small group did have an effect. It was very unnerving. It speaks to your own mortality, and that nothing in life is a given. It hurt the group because we never dealt adequately with their feelings about it. So I think that

there's an unresolved mourning issue that most of the group members are totally unaware of.

> [Female, 25 years practice, 20 years in PSG]

We had a death, and that was traumatic on every level, individually and groupwise. Other than that it's a very stable group, which is one of its great qualities.

> [Female, 20 years practice, 12 years in PSG]

There are some departures that are due to conflict, often because the issue isn't addressed or resolved. We will discuss how groups process (or fail to process) conflict in *Has there ever been overt conflict?* below.

In the five years I've been there two people left because there was an acrimonious personal interaction.

> [Male, 15 years practice, 5 years in PSG]

One person left in a state of feeling unsupported and criticized, and when we spoke with each other outside the group after her departure we expressed concern about her overall health, her mental health, but it wasn't discussed in the group. The other person left because there had been some overall displeasure with her by the women in the group prior to my joining.

> [Male, 40 years practice, 15 years in PSG]

But many groups are remarkably stable, some meeting for fifteen or twenty years without anyone leaving or being added.

A few people have come and gone over the years, but there is a core of people who have been there for at least fifteen years.

> [Male, 30 years practice, 25 years in PSG]

There is a core group that is the same as when I joined. A couple of people have come and gone, but it's pretty much the same group.

> [Female, 25 years practice, 15 years in PSG]

There was some turnover for the first ten years, people would come and go, but for the past ten years it's been the three of us.

> [Male, 45 years practice, 20 years in PSG]

## My own experience

My own group has been extremely stable. One man, a founding member in the group over thirty years, died suddenly last year, and the group is still adjusting to that loss. In a curious coincidence, we had already asked a new man to join the group when the founding member died. His death would have left me as the only man in the group, if not for the new member.

Outside of those two changes the group has remained the same for about fifteen years. Prior to that, there were several people who came into and left the group after a short time. The stability is important to me as it provides something we can all count on from week to week. I also like the lack of turnover because a new member destabilizes the group temporarily, and people are not as open and candid while feeling out the new person.

## Do the men function differently from the women?

There are stereotypes about men and women: men are more aggressive; women are more nurturing; men are more direct; women are more careful not to wound. This question tries to explore whether there are gender differences in the way people function in the group. The interviewees were equally divided on this question, with fifteen people saying that there were noticeable differences and fifteen saying there were none. (Four people were in groups of only one gender.)

Of those who saw differences, some saw them in general terms.

I do find men more direct, less worried about each other's feelings, which I find totally refreshing and nice, but also sometimes a little scary.

[Female, 25 years practice, 11 years in PSG]

I think this is a stereotype but I also think it's true: the women are more emotional, react more emotionally, and the man is not as likely to.

[Female, 35 years practice, 32 years in PSG]

One of the men is more assertive in saying that he wants to make certain points and wants to speak, and feels more comfortable doing that than the others do. So maybe there's a difference in terms of gender with the men being more assertive and aggressive.

[Female, 30 years practice, 30 years in PSG]

The biggest difference is that the men are less likely to want to get into their personal stuff. I don't mean countertransference, because that's really appropriate. I mean personal stuff that doesn't fit into our mission, our purpose.

[Female, 25 years practice, 20 years in PSG]

In our group it was very noticeable that the men stuck to the task and didn't get sidetracked, and were pragmatic and practical in their thinking.

[Female, 30 years practice, 3 years in PSG]

Every now and then the subgroupings emerge. If there's an issue about gender in the clinical focus, sometimes the men will find themselves having similar reactions, and there will be comments about the men versus the women.

[Male, 40 years practice, 15 years in PSG]

It's cultural. They have different perspectives. Women focus more on intimacy and the journey traveled together. Women are more aware of the importance of the power differential in relationships. For men, it's more of a focus on goal attainment and a tendency for competitiveness.

[Male, 45 years practice, 20 years in PSG]

Others saw differences in specific situations.

There's a married couple in the group, and the woman seems a little competitive with her husband sometimes, challenges him all the time. And she is confrontational with another member who's a friend outside the group.

[Female, 30 years practice, 8 months in PSG]

When someone brings up a sex issue, one of the men will start to make jokes. That then triggers the other group members, and we're going to have a little thing around it. Or they go off running in some weird direction, when it's not the focus of my problem. It's merely something I'm including, and people get stuck on it.

[Female, 25 years practice, 15 years in PSG]

I see differences only when we're talking about sexual issues. Because there you can see that the perspectives are somewhat different, and we sort of enlighten each other.

[Female, 35 years practice, 15 years in PSG]

One man added another variable of straight men versus gay men.

That's an interesting question because the women in the group are all straight. One of the men is straight and the other two are a gay couple. And the other difference is that the women and the gay couple are all psychologists, and the straight man is a psychiatrist, so there are significant differences. So it's more the five of us and him, rather than the men and the women. The five of us function in fairly similar ways: we tune into our experience, our thoughts and feelings in the room and in

our group. We touch on existential issues. We're supportive of one
another, very supportive and quite encouraging and caring and impressed with one another's work, and at the same time pointing out
what might be being overlooked or missed, or where the weak spot or
blind spot might be.

[Male, 15 years practice, 1 year in PSG]

The rest either saw no significant differences, or attributed them to the
character of the individuals, rather than their gender.

I'm not sure, because there have always been much fewer men. The
men have always been quite vocal, but I wonder if they might be listened to more because there are fewer of them.

[Female, 35 years practice, 30 years in PSG]

The men in this group tend to be very soft-spoken. I'm not sure that's a
gender difference.

[Male, 15 years practice, 5 years in PSG]

In cases that involve sexual abuse, I almost feel like I'm instructing this
one man, because he doesn't have that experience, and he's not able to
see the signs of it, or ask the right questions. It's not a gender thing.

[Female, 20 years practice, 15 years in PSG]

It's hard to know if it's gender or just personality. The man tends not to
initiate, he has to be invited.

[Female, 35 years practice, 5 years in PSG]

Sometimes it's because of this man's training. He's a psychologist who
does testing, and the training for a psychologist is different from that
for a social worker. So he has a very good perspective that the others,
who are both social workers, would not have thought of. Sometimes
it's because he doesn't have enough training, for example, any couples
case that involves sexual problems. He's skittish about that. I don't
think that's gender. That's just him as a person.

[Female, 20 years practice, 15 years in PSG]

One woman from a group consisting of seven women and only two men
suggested that, although differences had not emerged, that didn't mean
they weren't there.

## My own experience

I don't see much difference between the men and the women in my own
group. Of course there are differences, but I see them as individual and

not gender based. Because there are only two men, I find it difficult to generalize about men or women in the context of the group.

I tend to be outspoken and have strong opinions, and someone else might attribute some of that to my being a man, but there are several women in the group just as assertive and outspoken as I am. If I see any difference, I would say that it shows up as the women being more careful about how they phrase things, about trying more consciously not to hurt or offend.

## Discussion

Without question, private practice is isolating. It is so important to find some way to meet regularly with colleagues to relieve some of that isolation. It can also be a place for continuing education, and keeping up with new developments in the field. Although it's not a therapy group, it can be a forum for ongoing personal growth, as one understands better and better one's own blind spots and sensitive buttons.

I think it can take a few tries to find the right group. There are advantages and disadvantages to both joining an existing group and starting a group from scratch. In a new group, the founding members may determine who else they ask to join, what the rules and structure will be, and the time and place of meetings. Everyone is equal, and there are no preexisting conditions to deal with. People joining a group that has been already meeting have to find a way to fit in, but the advantage is that the group has had time to find its way and arrive at some stability.

People must know at least one person in the group or they would not have asked or been asked to join. Knowing many of the other members may make it easier to settle in and feel safe enough to present one's work. Depending on the size of the group, it may take a while for trust to develop.

There are advantages to having a lot of diverse backgrounds and theoretical orientations; different opinions and points of view can help see the case in a deeper way. Some people found that too many opinions were confusing, and theories and orientations too different from their own were not helpful (see Chapter 6: Presenting a Case).

Some groups have a lot of turnover, and some groups are incredibly stable. If a group has a lot of attrition, I would wonder what issues are not being addressed. For some people it's easier to leave the group than bring up their hurt, disappointment, or anger.

It's hard to generalize about gender differences. So often the differences we see in a group are particular to the individuals, not necessarily because they are one gender or another. What if we accept that men function differently from women? There are advantages to being direct, but also to being protective of others' feelings. It would seem to argue for making sure that there are both men and women in the group for optimal functioning.

I wonder about the people who are in more than one group now, and why they would limit the discussion to a narrow topic. On the other hand, peer group can be such a positive experience, why not have as much as possible?

We share a
→ Theoretical Orientation

# Chapter 5

# The Structure of the Group

In this chapter we will look at the way the group runs: what are the rules or agreements, understandings, and processes that give the group its structure. We might think of these aspects as the skeleton of the group, the frame that gives it shape and allows it to function.

These questions are pretty straightforward and in general don't evoke a lot of strong feelings. People do have reactions to some aspects, such as absences, or social contacts, but mostly these topics relate more to facts than to feelings.

## How often and how long do you meet? Does that feel like enough time?

Groups met weekly (seven), every two weeks (fifteen), or monthly (twelve), for meeting times of an hour (one), hour and a quarter (two), hour and a half (twenty-one), or two hours or more (ten).

More members said they were satisfied with the amount of time (twenty-two) than said they wanted more time (twelve). It had nothing to do with how often or how long they met—people whose group met once a week were just as likely to want more time as those who met monthly.

These statements are from people who met weekly.

We always feel short of time and rushed.
> [Female, 25 years practice, 11 years in PSG]

An hour and a half would be better [than seventy-five minutes]. It depends on the case we're discussing. Sometimes it's enough time, but if it's a very complicated case we feel like we need more time.
> [Female, 35 years practice, 15 years in PSG]

Some of those who met every other week wanted more time, not in more frequent meetings, but a longer session time.

It's never enough time.
> [Female, 5 years practice, 1 year in PSG]

It probably would be better if it were two full hours.
> [Female, 40 years practice, 17 years in PSG]

The members of the groups that met monthly often said that it was not enough time, but schedule commitments made meeting more often impractical.

If I didn't have my other groups I'd like it to meet more frequently but, given our schedules, that's what we could do. The personal group meets every week.
> [Female, 35 years practice, 2 years in PSG]

In terms of the functioning of the group, it would be useful to have more time, either more frequent meetings or more time. In terms of drain on my life space, it's enough.
> [Male, 15 years practice, 1 year in PSG]

This person found a solution.

It's not enough time but I fill in between by getting together in dyads.
> [Female, 10 years practice, 6 years in PSG]

Here's an interesting variation from someone whose group meets every two weeks for ninety minutes.

It feels just right. Or the group has trained me to think that it's the right time, I don't know.
> [Female, 25 years practice, 15 years in PSG]

## My own experience

My own group meets every other week for an hour and a half, and I like that alternate weeks I have a free block of time for personal errands or other activities. When I have a crisis with a patient, I wish we met more frequently and I didn't have to wait that extra week.

Sometimes the hour and a half goes too quickly and I wish we met longer. There are occasionally days when everyone has something to discuss and we run out of time before we all have a chance to present. Very rarely, the meeting drags and I wish we were done for the day. Most often, ninety minutes feels like just the right amount of time.

# Where do you meet?

Groups have the option of meeting consistently in one place or rotating meetings among the membership. The great majority (twenty-nine) met in the same place, usually a centrally located office. Meetings are only in another location when that person is away. A few people mentioned some of the particulars.

> Usually it's in one colleague's home. She has a big table that we sit around, and the person who's presenting brings the food, a coffee-and-snack kind of thing.
>
> [Female, 35 years practice, 15 years in PSG]

> I like the fact that it's here in my office, and nobody seems to mind. People come from all over and I'm very pleased. I'm very easy about having company. I don't get anxious about having people over.
>
> [Female, 30 years practice, 30 years in PSG]

Only a few (five) people said their groups rotate meeting places.

> It varies from coffee shops to someone's home or office.
>
> [Male, 10 years practice, 6 months in PSG]

> We rotate among the eight of us. We used to have what I called "The Great American Cook-off" because it became a cooking extravaganza, and the group lost the focus. The person who's hosting it provides some food now. We toned it down.
>
> [Female, 25 years practice, 20 years in PSG]

Even when the meeting space is unchanging, there are exceptions.

> On holidays or special occasions we meet in a restaurant.
>
> [Female, 35 years practice, 30 years in PSG]

## My own experience

I like that my own group almost always meets in the same office. If we have to relocate, I'm likely to forget and show up at the usual place, then have to run to the substitute location. I think having a regular venue contributes to the feeling of stability I get from the group.

My first peer group met in my own office, which was centrally located for the members. It certainly was easier not to have to travel, but I think I prefer going somewhere else that I don't have to straighten up after everyone leaves.

# Does the group have any sort of contract?

It's somewhat surprising that many (if not most) groups never discuss the contract—agreements about how the group will function. This was a typical description.

> When I joined it was "Welcome to the group." And subsequently people have left and joined but it's never discussed.
> [Male, 15 years practice, 5 years in PSG]

One person explained it this way.

> We all have the same orientation so we understand the agreements.
> [Female, 35 years practice, 5 years in PSG]

Confidentiality is often assumed, and for experienced professionals that is a given.

> Of course there's confidentiality. We totally trust each other, because we've known each other for so long. We didn't even have to say it.
> [Female, 35 years practice, 15 years in PSG]

> I don't think that there's a formal contract. It's understood that we don't talk to anyone outside the group. We've all been in the field long enough so that's kind of in our blood. We don't have to verbalize that.
> [Female, 40 years practice, 17 years in PSG]

> We have concerns about confidentiality, of course, and periodically we have to discuss that because someone is working with a patient that someone in the group might know.
> [Female, 25 years practice, 11 years in PSG]

There's an implicit agreement of confidentiality, especially since some of the members discuss their personal issues. And there's confidentiality about patients—we usually don't give their full name.

[Female, 35 years practice, 30 years in PSG]

I think there's a contract of confidentiality when we speak about a patient. And that's it. I guess there's a contract to show up, to be there as much as we can.

[Female, 30 years practice, 30 years in PSG]

People are thoughtful and even careful about how they give feedback about cases being presented, but this too is rarely discussed, unless someone objects to the way they are being spoken to.

There's a commitment, an understanding, that people will come to meetings, listen and be there for each other.

[Female, 20 years practice, 12 years in PSG]

Implicit agreements would be to try to understand whoever is presenting the case, their position, and, with what we know about them, to try to gently and constructively criticize.

[Female, 35 years practice, 32 years in PSG]

I think there are implicit agreements that we will help one another. We will talk about how the work affects us in addition to doing the clinical presentations.

[Female, 20 years practice, 15 years in PSG]

The unspoken rule is that everyone is respectful of everyone else, and if they have a problem with something that's going on or the way it's being said they often speak up right away. I don't think there's any holding back about that. The rule is "Whoever needs the time the most gets it."

[Female, 30 years practice, 30 years in PSG]

We agree that we're going to be as open and honest as we can.

[Male, 40 years practice, 7 years in PSG]

I think there's a kind of contract of kindness. I don't feel there's permission to be very aggressive. I think people have agreed to be polite, and I appreciate that, because it makes me feel safer.

[Female, 25 years practice, 15 years in PSG]

This group was very conscious of how they used the time.

We organized a group in which we would each spend twenty minutes talking about cases. Someone would be the timekeeper. And it pretty much worked that way. We might go over, but everyone would be respectful of ending and winding down on time.

[Female, 5 years practice, 1 year in PSG]

## Some groups negotiated the contract very explicitly and carefully.

We negotiated in the beginning what we wanted out of the group, we spoke about that. There were a couple of differences that were sticking points. One person wanted to talk about readings now and then, or suggest a reading. Two of the members were less inclined to focus on readings because they're in other groups where they do that, so they were more interested in talking about patients and issues. We resolved that everyone had that goal, but if one or two of us felt that it would be interesting to read something we could go ahead and do that and integrate it into the work, make it part of a clinical presentation.

[Female, 25 years practice, 1 year in PSG]

The criteria for membership became an explicit contract: that we would discuss our own groups as honestly and openly as possible, but we would also be open to issues of parallel process and to issues that occurred in the group, and be willing to address those and be willing to offer feedback to one another.

[Female, 35 years practice, 2 years in PSG]

All of us got together and actually drew up the contract. There were 8 specific agreements: 1) we will use the dialectical approach and respect each other's uniqueness; 2) we will use a consultant approach to the individual and help the person to help him- or herself, and we will avoid intervening on behalf of the patient unless we think it would be harmful not to, and we will discuss it with the group first; 3) members agree to respect individual differences—there is no right or wrong point of view; 4) we agree to be empathic and nonjudgmental with the patient; 5) we agree that everyone makes mistakes and we will be compassionate and nonjudgmental with each other; 6) we value individual differences; 7) we agree to attend each group, strive for punctuality, and inform the group of expected absences. Tardiness of over 5 minutes will be addressed and a behavioral analysis will occur within the group as well as a repair by doing a DBT-related activity; 8) we will experience gratitude for the training and each other. Someone was assigned the role of listening for any judgmental statements, and they had to ring a bell, and then there would be a discussion. The judgmental nuances could be as subtle as describing something as "resistance." Instead, we were supposed to use the term "therapy-interfering behavior."

[Female, 30 years practice, 3 years in PSG]

This description is of a peer supervision group that deals almost exclusively with therapy groups, not individual patients or couples.

> I don't think there's anything that's explicit in the sense that we negotiated, that we said that this is how we're going to function, or these are the kinds of things we're going to talk about. Or that we're going to keep everything confidential. Some of the people had been in other groups previously, and so had a kind of vision of what they wanted, and also knew what they didn't want. For example, one person said that they didn't want it to be over a meal, because in their past experience that turned it into a social experience. So while tea and cookies are often sitting there, that's not what it's about. That came from one person and everyone else agreed. I would say that there are understandings that are evolving. They're sort of explicit because they're talked about, but they're evolving with the process. One thing is that when people are talking about individual patients or if we're talking about the group process, someone is likely to bring it back to the groups that we're leading. That it's actually about consulting on our group psychotherapy work, not so much about our individual therapy work.
>
> [Male, 15 years practice, 1 year in PSG]

In some cases particular aspects of group functioning were addressed explicitly.

> We recently talked about having a "Keeper of the Space," whose job it is to keep the space clear for the person who's talking. If someone else is talking too it's their job to get their attention and remind them that the floor is taken.
>
> [Female, 25 years practice, 8 years in PSG]

## My own experience

In the peer group I organized, our contract was very brief and rather vague—only that we would discuss whatever cases we wanted to bring in. Coming in to an existing group I never learned if there ever was a contract or agreement. I was too busy trying to fit in to even think about it, although asking what the agreements were might have helped me do that.

As people joined after me, no one asked what the agreements were, and none were ever explained. I suspect that it might have made it easier and faster for us to settle in if we had been told what the contract was, rather than watching and observing and trying to deduce it on our own.

# How does the group normally begin?

After meeting for a while, often for many years, groups settle into a routine. As we mentioned before, agreements about group format are rarely discussed, but every group has a normal pattern.

Most people (twenty-two) said that the first few minutes are devoted to exchange of personal data, catching up with each other. Most people said they enjoyed this part of the meeting.

> Over the years it has become consistent that it begins with personal exchanges about what's happening in our lives, and follow-ups of that—health crises, and so on. We're very aware of each other's personal lives.
>
> [Male, 40 years practice, 15 years in PSG]

> There is usually some exchange of personal information, personal events and health updates and the like. Sometimes there is discussion of politics and other significant news events.
>
> [Male, 30 years practice, 25 years in PSG]

> It begins with at least one person being late, sometimes me. And there's usually a little bit of personal checking in. I think most of us like each other. It's while we're waiting for everyone to gather. When everyone has arrived, or it's clear that someone is going to be significantly late, someone will say, "Well, I have something I'd like to talk about."
>
> [Male, 15 years practice, 1 year in PSG]

But a few people said they didn't like the personal stuff, especially when it took up time better spent on clinical case material.

> At this point it begins by people finding out how everyone is, talking about the illnesses of their spouses, and at times I think we do that too much. When I've raised that issue, people have come down on me.
>
> [Female, 35 years practice, 30 years in PSG]

> It got worse and worse, and I had to exercise my role as the Supervision Nazi, and I said, "Listen, we're wasting a half hour talking about personal issues." Some people were very happy with that but I wasn't. Normally now somebody will say, "I have a case to present."
>
> [Female, 25 years practice, 20 years in PSG]

One group found a way to contain the personal material.

> The first fifteen minutes was schmooze time. The host would provide coffee and muffins, and was responsible for saying, "Okay, why don't

we get down to business now." The host would never be the presenter. So you didn't have double duty of having to prepare your presentation and having to host the meeting.

> [Female, 40 years practice, 15 years in PSG]

A smaller number (eight) said the group usually began with a case. Sometimes the person who presented was decided in advance. Even in a very structured group there can be personal conversation first.

> The person who's presenting that week, they know in advance. We decided that we're going in alphabetical order by first names. The person goes twice and then the next person goes twice, unless somebody's on vacation or sick, and then we skip them and then we go back to them. So we usually start by chatting for about three minutes, socially, and then the person starts.
>
> [Female, 35 years practice, 15 years in PSG]

> There are a couple of people who function as leaders without being designated as such, and they'll say, "Does anyone have a case?" Usually we try to have two cases and one issue. Sometimes it's established by email before we meet.
>
> [Male, 10 years practice, 3 years in PSG]

> Usually we know who's presenting because we address that at the end of the previous meeting. Somebody has something that they're struggling with that they're concerned about, and it's timely, so they want to bring that in for the next session. So they come with notes, and maybe the file.
>
> [Female, 25 years practice, 1 year in PSG]

Four people said the group began in a different way.

> In the beginning it was very structured, and we would begin with a mindfulness exercise. One person would be assigned the role of leader, and one the role of observer. The observer would alert the group when any of the agreements were being broken. The leader could determine the structure of the group for that day. Leadership would rotate, and we would take the role for a month at a time.
>
> [Female, 30 years practice, 3 years in PSG]

> We open with a short meditation.
>
> [Female, 10 years practice, 6 years in PSG]

> First we order food.
>
> [Male, 10 years practice, 6 months in PSG]

I send out emails every month as a reminder, and I set the agenda. We usually start with some kind of chitchat about something that's going on, a conference that some people went to, something external to the group, and then we begin to move into what our agenda is.

[Female, 30 years practice, 8 months in PSG]

### My own experience

My group always begins with some social small talk and personal announcements. There are nine members, and it never happens that everyone arrives at once, so we need to fill the time until everyone is there. There's no point in beginning a case presentation if people are going to trickle in and the presenter has to go back over the material again.

Because these are people who are important in my life, I want to fill them in on any significant developments, and want to know what's going on in their lives, too. This beginning time gives us all a chance to exchange this information.

## Are there any fees involved?

A peer group implies to me that no one is being paid as the leader or the "expert." In most situations there was no exchange of money. A few groups did buy food or beverages for the meeting. Sometimes the expenses are shared.

We pay the person whose house it is for providing the coffee.

[Female, 35 years practice, 15 years in PSG]

One person buys lunch every week, and that rotates.

[Female, 20 years practice, 7 years in PSG]

Other times the host is not reimbursed.

Someone provides snacks.

[Male, 45 years practice, 5 years in PSG]

Whoever hosts it just provides.

[Female, 35 years practice, 2 years in PSG]

People bring lunch and I serve soda or tea or something for them.

[Female, 35 years practice, 30 years in PSG]

The treats are provided by the person in whose place we're meeting.

[Male, 15 years practice, 1 year in PSG]

A few people mentioned other kinds of financial arrangements.

> When it's the full group we rent the space and chip in for that.
> [Female, 10 years practice, 6 years in PSG]

> We each put in twenty dollars a session, and we have a treasurer. We're probably going to get a website, and maybe do some advertising, and this money will pay for that.
> [Female, 30 years practice, 8 months in PSG]

This person thought the fact that peer supervision doesn't involve payment to a group leader was a problem.

> I think that's why the group died, because we weren't accountable financially.
> [Female, 5 years practice, 1 year in PSG]

**My own experience**
In my group, we don't pay for anything. There's normally nothing to pay for. On special occasions, weddings, birthdays, and such, we may buy a gift and all chip in.

# Do you discuss your personal lives?

Only two people said their group never discusses the personal lives of the members. Often there is the social interaction at the beginning of the meeting, and sometimes personal issues become relevant when discussing a countertransference problem. This is a typical response.

> There are a lot of friends in the group and a casualness about relating the issue and how it impacts them personally. It's still kept very focused on the issue, but some personal information is brought in.
> [Male, 10 years practice, 3 years in PSG]

For some people exchange of personal information is an important aspect of the group.

> We would talk about crisis in someone's life. Personal crisis: health, children, anything, and that always takes precedence.
> [Female, 25 years practice, 15 years in PSG]

> Normally, we report significant events. People occasionally discuss things like difficulty with a spouse or a child, or health issues and such.
> [Male, 30 years practice, 25 years in PSG]

People are aware that a lot of social conversation may shift the focus of the group in an unwanted way.

> When anything major is going on with somebody we hear about it. We don't necessarily discuss everything that's making us anxious, but for the most part we do mention the major issues. We try not to use it as a therapy group.
>
> [Female, 40 years practice, 17 years in PSG]

> We probably keep very personal stuff out of the group. There are certain kinds of problems that I wouldn't bring to the group. But I might discuss them with some of the people in the group outside of the group.
>
> [Female, 20 years practice, 7 years in PSG]

> Occasionally if someone's been going through some gruesome thing we'll spend some time on that, but we never take the whole meeting.
>
> [Female, 25 years practice, 11 years in PSG]

When the social chatting starts to intrude into the clinical time, adjustments may be made.

> Initially we met in someone's home, and food would be brought. We decided that there was too much socializing, too much personal material at the front of the group, which didn't leave enough time for the clinical material. We agreed to cut down the socializing and focus on the clinical material.
>
> [Male, 15 years practice, 5 years in PSG]

When the topic elicits personal reactions, it can be useful to reveal them to the group.

> We did where it was relevant, where it had to do with therapy-interfering behavior on the therapist's part. Or if the patient was evoking a certain kind of response you might do a behavior analysis, in which you would try to identify what the precipitating events or vulnerabilities were. If someone is reminding you of someone in your life, and that's triggering some kind of reaction in you, then you would look at it.
>
> [Female, 30 years practice, 3 years in PSG]

> Sometimes it's clearly an issue of transference and countertransference—those are the most interesting. We can discuss it because we feel so safe with each other. We don't go into long diatribes on a personal basis, but we may be reminded of something from our past and we can talk about it there, and see the parallel, and it's very helpful.
>
> [Female, 20 years practice, 15 years in PSG]

It's inevitable, when you're talking about topics like money, that you're going to be talking about your personal life: my difficulties and challenges in bringing my fee where I'd like it to be; how I went from one fee to another fee; my recognition that I'm a competent professional providing something of value; how that relates to the fees that you get and the boundaries that you set; how you formulate your policies, like with cancellations. There's an interface between personal and professional.

[Male, 10 years practice, 6 months in PSG]

Sometimes the conversation turns personal in an unexpected way.

One time, and this never happened again, someone was getting certified in addiction treatment, and we spent the whole time talking about our personal drug use, as teenagers and so on.

[Female, 25 years practice, 11 years in PSG]

**My own experience**
My group does discuss our personal lives, and for most of us it's an important aspect of being in the group. We know each other a very long time, and are important people in each other's lives, both personal and professional. Weddings (our own and our children's), divorces, illnesses and recoveries, professional accomplishments, vacation trips, and such, are all mentioned and discussed.

For me, it deepens the experience of being with these people, week after week, year after year. I can't imagine not wanting to tell them about the important milestones in my life.

# Do members socialize? How do you think that affects the functioning of the group?

Only four of the interviewees said their group did not socialize with each other, although several others said they didn't socialize themselves but at least some of the rest of the group did see each other socially. For many people the social contacts in the group were a natural and normal part of their personal lives.

Two of the people are very close friends and see each other a lot. Two of the people I see a lot because we're part of the same institute.

[Female, 25 years practice, 11 years in PSG]

The group is usually invited to significant events like weddings, parties, and such. Some people are friends outside of the group.

[Male, 30 years practice, 25 years in PSG]

Together as a group, once every year or two we have a dinner, and we invite our significant others and we've done that five or six times over the eleven years.

[Female, 25 years practice, 11 years in PSG]

Unlike therapy groups, there is normally no rule forbidding outside contact.

I live with one of them, so we socialize all the time. I know that some of the others do. There's certainly no agreement that we won't do that.

[Male, 15 years practice, 1 year in PSG]

Groups had different ways of managing these relationships.

Sometimes someone will say, "I've already talked to so-and-so about this," and then they'll fill the rest of the group in.

[Female, 25 years practice, 11 years in PSG]

It's kind of acknowledged that when we tell the group about something personal, some people know already.

[Female, 25 years practice, 11 years in PSG]

I do socialize with one person in the group but it doesn't feel like it interferes with the group's functioning. We do not gossip, though, about the group. I wouldn't be comfortable with that without bringing it back to the group.

[Female, 25 years practice, 1 year in PSG]

Every now and then there'll be a reference to a conversation that a dyad had outside the group, something related to a patient, and they're very quick to bring the rest of us up to date.

[Male, 40 years practice, 15 years in PSG]

In some groups people are careful about maintaining the boundaries.

One of the people is a very good friend who lives nearby, and the closeness of that relationship has enhanced the peer group for both of us, but we don't talk about the peer group outside the group. When I socialize with any of the group members I don't talk about the peer group.

[Female, 35 years practice, 2 years in PSG]

Many people saw socializing as a normal part of the life of the group.

In some ways I think it helps the group to function that there are at least some relationships that are already trusting, and have a history and a common language. I think it highlights that some people don't have as close a connection as others, but we're all experienced enough as people and as group therapists to recognize that that's life and that's how groups work, and we try to manage that.

[Male, 20 years practice, 1 year in PSG]

Some people saw minimal effect on the group, even when there was obvious tension.

The group is very open with each other about our cases and our experience in the group and the outside contact doesn't seem to affect that.

[Female, 35 years practice, 15 years in PSG]

I think that two or three of the group members do have lunch together. They're very honest and open about it so I don't think it affects the group.

[Male, 40 years practice, 7 years in PSG]

I think there was a little tension. Another woman and I had been exercise partners, and we had a falling out that I've never understood. She and her husband would get together with the other woman in the group and her husband for holidays, and the third woman was close with the wife of one of the men. It just caused a little tension but I don't think it interfered with the group's functioning.

[Female, 40 years practice, 15 years in PSG]

I do socialize with several of them, and that preceded the existence of the group. I don't see much effect.

[Female, 25 years practice, 8 years in PSG]

Some people thought the social aspect of the group enhanced the functioning of the group.

Some of the socializing of the group as a whole at different shared events, like weddings, has felt like it builds group cohesion.

[Female, 25 years practice, 15 years in PSG]

Unlike a therapy group where we don't encourage socialization, as clinicians it's helpful to know who it is we're working with, referring to, and opening up our clinical material to. It can actually deepen the experience.

[Male, 15 years practice, 5 years in PSG]

I think it can be a positive thing, because you get more acquainted personally with people in the group.

[Male, 40 years practice, 8 months in PSG]

We socialize more with some than with others. We meet at least twice a year at group dinners where we drink and eat. I think that it enhances group functioning.

[Female, 25 years practice, 15 years in PSG]

Others saw problems resulting from the social contact.

Some people socialized, and that conversation would spill over into the group. We had a hard time staying with the task.

[Female, 35 years practice, 2 years in PSG]

It stirs up feelings of envy or competition within the group at times. Are people being protective of the relationships they have formed? Am I going to call someone on their lack of clinical acumen?

[Male, 15 years practice, 5 years in PSG]

I sometimes feel a little left out, even though I know I leave myself out.

[Female, 40 years practice, 18 years in PSG]

There are subgroups, people who see each other outside of group, and that takes up group time, pairing off and having conversations, and it takes away from the energy of the group.

[Female, 25 years practice, 8 years in PSG]

I think that it does change the nature of the group that some people socialize more than others, but since some are longstanding friends this seems unavoidable and intrinsic to this group. Besides, I like that there are not too many rules to follow.

[Female, 20 years practice, 12 years in PSG]

People can feel excluded from the closer relationships that others have developed.

Some people might feel more like outsiders. I think it's subtle, but it exists.

[Male, 10 years practice, 3 years in PSG]

When I think of one person in the group in particular, I have the sense that she is not happy that I haven't reached out to her and socialized more. That hurts her feelings and makes her angry, and so things are kept very superficial between us. We were closer at one time, but I felt the friendship diminishing, and I had less time and less interest in pursuing it.

[Female, 30 years practice, 30 years in PSG]

> I think it may leave some people feeling more like an outsider some-
> times.
>
> [Male, 30 years practice, 25 years in PSG]

People can be selective about what they reveal to whom.

> We probably keep very personal stuff out of the group. There are cer-
> tain kinds of problems that I wouldn't bring to the group. But I might
> discuss them with some of the people in the group outside of the group.
>
> [Female, 20 years practice, 7 years in PSG]

One person mentioned that the effect depends on the content of what is
discussed outside the group.

> I don't think socializing affects the group adversely unless group issues
> are discussed which would be better handled by the group.
>
> [Female, 45 years practice, 30 years in PSG]

### My own experience

Some of the people in my group have been friends forever, even before
they joined the group, so they see each other outside of group all the
time. Others have met in the group and like each other well enough to
want to get together socially, both with and without partners.

I would hate to have a rule that we were not allowed to socialize,
because that would feel infantilizing. I don't see personal relationships
interfering with group functioning in my own group, although I can see
how such situations could arise.

# How do absences affect the group?

Inevitably, people are sometimes away from group: illness, vacation,
emergencies with patients, and so on. These absences have effects on the
group process and on the individual members. Many people had strong
reactions to other members being absent.

> One or two people are frequently absent. I think it's destructive to the
> group. The group has learned to accommodate it, but I don't think it's
> good for the group at all. It undermines the purpose of the group. It can
> feel at times like it's derailing the group.
>
> [Female, 25 years practice, 15 years in PSG]

It's better when people come regularly, that you can count on them,
that there's a sense of commitment from them. When people don't

come regularly, there's a sense of not feeling important, that the group isn't that important.

[Female, 20 years practice, 12 years in PSG]

One of the women often calls in and says she didn't get enough sleep and isn't coming. I really don't like that. It moves us off what's relevant.

[Male, 45 years practice, 5 years in PSG]

People are often angry or resentful toward members who are consistently absent.

I feel less generous toward that person in terms of my willingness to give time and focus on their problems, because they come in and say "I have a case, let's do me," and I think, "How about all the other times when you weren't here?"

[Female, 30 years practice, 30 years in PSG]

There are certain people who are iffy in their attendance and it's annoying. I think we all find it annoying.

[Female, 30 years practice, 30 years in PSG]

A few specific people are consistently absent a lot. It can be a problem when they come back and want to commandeer the group because they have so much accumulated material. The group is large enough that even several absences still leave enough people present to have a meaningful interaction.

[Male, 30 years practice, 25 years in PSG]

A few people seemed to be able to shrug off their own reactions.

Some people are more absent than others. There's a temporary feeling of abandonment, and some anger, but when that person is here it doesn't seem to affect the group.

[Female, 40 years practice, 18 years in PSG]

Groups, especially when they are small, are affected when people are missing.

We miss the feedback from those people; we miss their participation. One person was going to do a presentation and we had to delay it because so many people were out.

[Female, 30 years practice, 8 months in PSG]

People are not absent often, but, since we are only five, an absent member is felt, since the feedback is not as rich. Some members are more talkative, and if that member is absent it is felt more strongly. There is one person who is a central character in the group and the person in whose house we meet. Her absence means we need to move the site of the group as well. Absences also mean that we have to rearrange presentation order, but that doesn't seem to affect us very much.

[Female, 35 years practice, 15 years in PSG]

The smaller group created by several absences can be a very different experience.

There are twelve members, but only six or seven show up for any given meeting. Usually it's a little bit of a relief that some people don't come, because we're so many. I've thought and said as much that it's nice when it's a smaller group. We've had groups as small as three, and it's still dynamic and stimulating. There's always a hope that it's a good turnout, but not much disappointment when some people don't turn up.

[Male, 10 years practice, 3 years in PSG]

There are frequently at least one or two people missing. Sometimes, a smaller group feels more intimate, and can have its advantages. Other times, people are missed.

[Female, 40 years practice, 17 years in PSG]

People who are more knowledgeable about and experienced with group functioning may be more careful about absences.

We were all group people, so we already had a concept of how groups should be. Everyone was very committed, and it was very rare for anyone to be absent for anything other than being sick or on vacation, which would get announced ahead of time.

[Female, 40 years practice, 15 years in PSG]

I think it interferes with a kind of accretion of ongoing understanding of the things we're talking about. And it also generates feelings that we then work with in the parallel process. It's useful material to work with, but ultimately it interferes and I don't think it serves the group process.

[Male, 15 years practice, 1 year in PSG]

Several people whose groups had terminated saw absences as a contributing factor.

It minimized the importance of the group. That's partially why it fizzled out. There were two people who would just flake out, and say, "I can't do it, it's not going to work for me," and really didn't make it a priority.

[Female, 5 years practice, 1 year in PSG]

It may be difficult to get the group to address the issue of how absences affect its functioning.

> I think it affects the trust in the group, I think it affects the continuity. It generates some angry feelings, and some hurt feelings that are not really processed. It has been brought up, but the group doesn't stay very well with its feelings.
>
> [Female, 25 years practice, 20 years in PSG]

> Attendance was an issue with one person, and that made it very difficult. It made constancy and consistency difficult. It made dealing with the interpersonal process much more difficult, because you couldn't be sure, if you opened an issue that dealt with the group itself, that you could count on that person being back the next time. As a result, when a hot issue came up that we hadn't anticipated, and somebody didn't come the next time, that was very problematic.
>
> [Female, 35 years practice, 2 years in PSG]

People who are absent can leave a hole that the group may have trouble filling.

> One woman was absent quite a bit, and very apologetic, very clear that she had good reasons. She knew when she joined that this would happen, and we talked a lot before she joined about whether to include her, that was one of the concerns. We love having her in the group, so it's not so much an issue. Sometimes someone will say, "I wish she was here, I miss her take on this."
>
> [Female, 25 years practice, 11 years in PSG]

One group had recently experienced the death of one of its members, and this permanent absence had affected everyone.

> When he spoke we all listened, so we're missing that. He had a certain way of saying things, and a certain expertise that is missed already.
>
> [Female, 35 years practice, 30 years in PSG]

> The groups after the funeral were strange—people talking about other things than the death, and having side conversations. It was making me crazy. It felt to me like orphans in an asylum, all very needy but not knowing how to ask for what we needed. There have been other times when people have been not there, but this time I felt bereft.
>
> [Female, 40 years practice, 17 years in PSG]

In some groups absences are considered normal and expectable.

Absences are the exception. It always elicits comments, how come, and what happened, I wanted to say something to him or her. On the other hand, I see it as part of reality and modern life.

[Male, 40 years practice, 7 years in PSG]

Absences have different kinds of effects on different groups.

It always has an effect on the group when a personality isn't there, but other things compensate for it, because other people have more of a chance to talk up.

[Female, 35 years practice, 30 years in PSG]

We know each other so well that we always miss the input of whoever's absent. We miss what they would say, and we gear what we're bringing up to who is there.

[Female, 25 years practice, 15 years in PSG]

Everybody's very committed to the group, so people don't like to miss, but sometimes things come up. If two people are out, the other two people will tend to go out for lunch and make it a social occasion.

[Female, 20 years practice, 7 years in PSG]

We might well meet anyway. They're missed but it doesn't stop the conversation.

[Male, 10 years practice, 6 months in PSG]

Absences, especially when consistent or when several members are out, can indicate anger about how the group is functioning.

The group functioned extremely well in the beginning, and then there was a change in the administration's policy toward the group. They had approved paying for the training, they gave us the time off for it, they gave us the time during the week for the group, and then after the training we decided that we wanted to hire an expert in DBT as a consultant. We were all going to chip in out of our own pockets as a team. At that point it became clear that this was something that was not supported by administrative policy, and that impacted on the group. After that, a lot of people were disheartened. Over the next year, people started losing interest in the treatment and in the group. The group grew smaller and smaller, until there were only three people left, and it soon after disbanded.

[Female, 30 years practice, 3 years in PSG]

**My own experience**

I am rarely absent from group. It's too important a part of my life to miss unless I have to. I miss meetings when I'm ill or out of town; otherwise I'm there.

   I am unhappy when other people are absent, even if they have a good explanation. The group feels diminished, even though we are large enough to have a group that feels full even when several people are missing. I can feel devalued by the absent person, and may not want to listen to them when they return. There are a few people who are often absent, and it makes me question their commitment.

# Do you read papers/books and discuss them?

Most people (twenty-three) said that their peer supervision group read articles at least occasionally; the others (eleven) said that they did not. Sometimes this was because they were in other situations in which they did their clinical reading, and sometimes it didn't seem to be a priority.

   Most of the members are in other groups where they read, or we're teaching so we have to read. I was in a writing group as well. Once in a while, if someone has a paper that they think is totally relevant to a case, we'll pass that around.
                               [Female, 25 years practice, 11 years in PSG]

   I used to do much more reading, especially when I was teaching. I was also in a reading group, so I got that somewhere else.
                               [Female, 35 years practice, 32 years in PSG]

   Not in this group, because I do that in another group. This group is purely supervision.
                               [Female, 35 years practice, 15 years in PSG]

Many people said they enjoy reading and discussing relevant articles, and consider it part of the work of the group.

   We read both books and papers. We complete assignments. Some of it is very helpful.
                               [Female, 30 years practice, 3 years in PSG]

   I find it stimulating. Often it's stuff that I had read before, but then I hear it in a new light.
                               [Female, 35 years practice, 30 years in PSG]

I collect conferences, papers, and so on, and I put them out when people arrive. If we go to a conference we would present that to the others.

[Female, 35 years practice, 30 years in PSG]

We do that all the time. It's part of the work.

[Female, 10 years practice, 6 years in PSG]

Some groups had tried including reading and discussing papers, but found that there was not enough interest to continue doing it.

I don't get the feeling that that's the major area of interest for the people in the group. It's been one a year, tops, maybe not even that.

[Female, 40 years practice, 17 years in PSG]

For a few years we met additionally once a month to read papers and books and discuss them. We all liked it but it was a lot of work. Periodically we say that we should start that again but we haven't. We probably will at some point.

[Female, 20 years practice, 7 years in PSG]

We've tried from time to time, but it never seems to catch on very much.

[Female, 45 years practice, 30 years in PSG]

Some people whose group did not often read articles or books wished that they did more often.

Sometimes someone will bring in an article or a book but it's rare. I brought in an article and they said, "That's nice." But we didn't discuss it. I wish they did. I miss it. I'm understimulated in the group.

[Male, 15 years practice, 5 years in PSG]

We would reference papers, and recommend papers. We wouldn't read them as a group or discuss them. We thought about doing it but we never did. I wish we had.

[Female, 5 years practice, 1 year in PSG]

I would like to, but there hasn't been much interest.

[Female, 35 years practice, 5 years in PSG]

Some others whose group did read and discuss articles wished they didn't spend time on it.

We've done that, but not very successfully. I don't particularly want it.

[Female, 25 years practice, 15 years in PSG]

We tried that at one point. Someone suggested a book about being a therapist, and we discussed a couple of chapters. I don't want more of that.

[Male, 10 years practice, 3 years in PSG]

We have occasionally read papers. I don't enjoy it and do it reluctantly. I feel like that is something I can do on my own.

[Male, 30 years practice, 25 years in PSG]

We tried that and it was not too successful. One person had suggested and we tried it and it didn't work. People really wanted to do less didactic and more clinical.

[Female, 25 years practice, 20 years in PSG]

Occasionally there is a group in which a member is an author.

There was an occasion where I had published a book that I wanted the group to read and discuss, and they had tremendous resistance to doing that. I was frustrated and hurt that they didn't seem to care.

[Male, 30 years practice, 25 years in PSG]

If someone in the group is writing something they'll share it with us, and we become a source of feedback to the author.

[Male, 40 years practice, 15 years in PSG]

## My own experience

I don't want to spend group time on books and papers that I can select and read myself. If I come across published material that's exciting and thought-provoking, I'll certainly tell the group about it and, if the others read it, then we may discuss it. But for me the group time is too valuable to spend it on papers and books.

# What is the structure of a typical meeting?

We described earlier how often groups begin with some personal chat, catching up with each other for ten or fifteen minutes. Then the clinical material is addressed. Groups do this in various ways. Some groups are fairly structured.

We normally start by setting up the next meeting first. Someone takes minutes and we go over the minutes, if there's anything left over from the previous meeting we address that. People have asked for time, that's actually done in advance of the meeting, when I send out the reminder. Then people present however they want to do it. We talk about

the issue; we talk about other cases that are similar. It's always a difficult case, and we give feedback.

[Female, 30 years practice, 8 months in PSG]

Someone knows they're going to present. If it's not a focused issue that
the therapist is having, it'll be presented as just the details around the
case and we'll all start to react, have questions, wonder out loud, and
things get going. If it's something someone is struggling with, then
they'll take a little more time to present what the clinical issues have
been, what the impasse is about, with some history of the client.

[Female, 25 years practice, 1 year in PSG]

There are a couple of people who function as leaders without being
designated as such, and they'll say, "Does anyone have a case?" Usually we try to have two cases and one issue. Sometimes it's established
by email before we meet. We try to structure it in terms of time, because sometimes it gets rambly when we talk about a case, and we'll
put a time limit on it.

[Male, 10 years practice, 3 years in PSG]

One person presents a case twice, two weeks in a row. They go back
and try what we've talked about, and then they come back and tell us
what happened, and get a little more. So it's really a follow-through
with deeper thinking about the case. Anytime, even between the first
and second presentation, if anyone has anything urgent, then they go. It
takes precedence.

[Female, 20 years practice, 15 years in PSG]

Sometimes we structure it using a Group as Expert model, where you
describe the case in a few minutes, and then ask a question, and then
each person says as the expert what they would do and how they would
view it. We might hire a consultant for a session to help us to deepen
our work.

[Female, 25 years practice, 8 years in PSG]

Most groups are more spontaneous.

First we check in with each other, and then someone will begin with a
case that's on their mind. There's no formal presentation and no rota-
tion of who presents. Someone says they have something they'd like to
talk about. We listen pretty intently to the presentation and then we in-
formally respond. We stay with that until it feels done, and then someone else will say they want to present something.

[Female, 20 years practice, 7 years in PSG]

The group doesn't rush a case or a presenter; we stay with it until they feel they've gotten what they need. We stay, sometimes the whole session, until the presenter feels a comfort level, which is a very graceful way to handle things. There's no sense that you better get on with it, pick this up fast because we want to get on to our own cases. People don't do that.

[Female, 20 years practice, 12 years in PSG]

We have a little socialization, and then somebody will bring up an issue, and we give that as much time as is required. Somebody might say, "I have a new patient and I'm confused about this or that, I need some feedback from the group" or "I think I'm having a countertransference reaction, please help." Sometimes it'll be a question about billing or insurance, a more general issue of private practice. Other people will join in and give their impressions. Sometimes it's a free-for-all. How long we spend on an issue varies. It's until the person feels satisfied. We might ask, "Did you get what you need?"

[Female, 45 years practice, 30 years in PSG]

After the chitchat, which lasts about ten minutes while people arrive, someone says "I have a case" or "I have something I need to discuss." We try to make sure there's enough time to accommodate everyone. People present the case in a very informal way; sometimes it's too unstructured and we have to ask the presenter what they want. People ask questions, make suggestions, and usually a consensus is reached about how to proceed.

[Male, 30 years practice, 25 years in PSG]

Usually there's a big case, and then some codas. Someone will present a case for about forty-five minutes and then one or two people will tag on a case that's similar that they may have had in their own practice that's related to the main issue. Someone presents and people interrupt, some more than others, and ask questions, and try to be helpful and be interpretive.

[Female, 20 years practice, 12 years in PSG]

One person saw the lack of formal structure as a potential problem.

It's pretty amorphous. It's based on urgency, on people's needs, and some people are better at expressing that than others. That can be a problem.

[Female, 40 years practice, 17 years in PSG]

One group went from more structured to less so.

> When the group first started, we started out rotating who presented, so we had a more formal structure where we took turns. At some point, when a member left the group and someone new joined, he questioned that, and we had a whole discussion about it and decided to try less structure. We discussed it again a few months later and decided that we all liked it better.
>
> [Female, 25 years practice, 11 years in PSG]

Presenters may ramble, and someone will try to help them focus.

> First we chat, and then someone says they have a case. They'll present the case. If they go on too long I tend to focus the group on what's the problem? Why are you bringing up this case? I'm good at that.
>
> [Female, 35 years practice, 30 years in PSG]

> If someone goes on for fifteen minutes in doing a presentation it's way too long. We would be asking them to frame the question. What do you want us to be paying attention to? We don't want the full history.
>
> [Female, 35 years practice, 2 years in PSG]

Time is divided and allocated among those who want to present.

> Depending on how many people want to present we divide the time, and say how much time they can present for.
>
> [Female, 25 years practice, 8 years in PSG]

> We'll look at what we have to do. One person will present a case, and people will ask questions. People will give their opinion along the way, and not wait until the end. Sometimes the presentation will have to do with a question that the presenter really needs answered. When we feel satisfied that we have some resolution, then we move on to the next person.
>
> [Female, 20 years practice, 15 years in PSG]

> To some degree there may be some self-monitoring, like "I spoke a lot last time. Does anybody else have something?" Or "I've been talking for a while. This is really helpful but I want to make space for others." Or someone saying, "I do want us to save some time for something I want to talk about." So there's an informal group-level negotiation about time. There certainly isn't a structure that everyone presents, or everyone speaks every time. It's much more informal.
>
> [Male, 15 years practice, 1 year in PSG]

Sometimes someone just jumps in and starts talking, and somewhere in the meeting the other person needs to say that they need some time. We don't have an explicit agenda, and we don't say that everybody gets 15 minutes. People remember that someone asked for time, even if they get caught up in something, and come back to that person. There's a gatekeeping, but it doesn't reside in any one person, which I think is a measure of a high-functioning peer group.

[Female, 35 years practice, 2 years in PSG]

We find out who has something they want to be sure to cover, and then we open it up from there. We divide the time as needed.

[Male, 10 years practice, 6 months in PSG]

Some groups try intentionally to divide the time.

We try to have at least two people present in the two hours.

[Female, 35 years practice, 32 years in PSG]

Usually everybody gets to talk about something. It's an extension of the principle in the modern analytic group that everyone takes their fair share of the time. We make sure that everyone gets to talk.

[Female, 35 years practice, 5 years in PSG]

And some groups try to stay with a single case.

Generally we would focus on the one case for the whole time. We would try to use any emotional reactions and any process we would experience in the room. But I think that's difficult in a leaderless group.

[Female, 40 years practice, 15 years in PSG]

Urgency almost always trumps any previous agreement about who is presenting.

Whoever has the most pressing issue gets to present.

[Female, 30 years practice, 3 years in PSG]

Someone will say, "I have a case," someone else will say, "Well, I have case, too," and whoever feels the most urgency gets to speak first.

[Female, 30 years practice, 30 years in PSG]

We'll talk about what's going on with us until everyone gathers. If there's one or two who are late, and it's urgent, whoever needs to start will start with whoever's there, even if it's only one person, and everyone else will catch up as they come in.

[Female, 25 years practice, 15 years in PSG]

It's set up so that whoever feels the most pressure to talk about something, or get help with a patient, gets to say that at the beginning, and we try to make time for that.

[Female, 25 years practice, 20 years in PSG]

People have different ways of making a case presentation.

One of the members always has notes, and an outline of what the session was, and he always passes it out so that we can follow along. I never do that. I just talk in terms of what my issue is, and tell them, remind them of the case. Some of us take notes during the presentation part, to remember, and some of us don't.

[Female, 35 years practice, 15 years in PSG]

Some groups ask the presenter to be clear about what he or she wants from the group.

Sometimes you have to ask what's bothering them about the case.

[Female, 25 years practice, 20 years in PSG]

They'll start off by saying "I'm distressed by this or that," or "I can't figure this out, " or "I feel guilty or upset or confused," and we start with having a sense of the reason for the presentation.

[Male, 40 years practice, 15 years in PSG]

Before the feedback begins we ask the presenter what his specific questions are, if they're clear to him. Sometimes they're not, and he just wants to get our impressions.

[Male, 10 years practice, 3 years in PSG]

Some groups leave time to examine the group process itself.

About every cycle, in which everyone would present once, we would have an open meeting where we talk about how we were as a group. Anyone could trump that if they had something urgent, but it was really helpful.

[Female, 40 years practice, 15 years in PSG]

In most groups, the presenter describes the patient and the situation that he or she wants help with. Here the presentation went a little differently.

A big part of the group was role-playing, so you actually got to watch how someone else worked. So if I'm in a stuck place with a patient, and I can play my patient really well, I can see how someone else would get unstuck.

[Female, 30 years practice, 3 years in PSG]

Several people highlighted the advantages of meeting with the same group of people over time.

> They may be working with a friend or relative of the patient being discussed, and so they may know some other information about the case and add a little more data.
>
> [Male, 40 years practice, 8 months in PSG]

> What I think often happens, and this gets to the core of why I think the group is so helpful, is that we know each other well enough now to know how our stuff comes up with patients. So that it doesn't take very long when someone's presenting something to get a sense of where the person's stuck because of their own history or their own issues. Countertransference issues get picked up very quickly, much more quickly than if we were dealing with people we didn't know well.
>
> [Female, 40 years practice, 17 years in PSG]

## My own experience

As I mentioned above, my group always begins with some personal updates. As people come in, they might say that they have something to present and would like some time. When everyone is there, people present in turn, and everyone else questions and comments until the presenters say that they have what they need.

Recently we began setting aside some time for group process, something we had done only occasionally in the past. This has been very interesting, and has for me added some depth and meaning that I felt was missing. So far, we have discussed some resentment one of the members was feeling, and looked at better ways of making a presentation.

# Discussion

In this section, we have looked at some of the arrangements and agreements that allow the group to function. I think of them as analogous to the frame of a building or the rules of a game.

Almost all groups begin with some social chat, catching up with each other. This helps establish reconnection, but can be frustrating if it goes on too long and takes too much time away from the clinical discussions. But I think it's important psychologically to reconnect before plunging into the case material. Also, if the group is going to understand a presenter's case, and the difficulty he or she is having with the patient, then members are going to have to reveal themselves as people. This includes both their current situations and their personal histories. It's so often the case that the therapist's history is at the root of his or her countertransferential reactions, and the group needs to know at least the broad outlines to be able to help.

The question of social contact outside the group is an interesting area of group functioning. Peer supervision groups are not therapy groups, and there are normally no rules against outside contact. Many of the members are friends outside of the group, and do socialize. This can lead to formation of subgroups, and at worst can interfere with group functioning. The group that addresses group process can deal with whatever problems come up as a result of outside social connections.

I was really surprised that so few people could articulate any sort of group contract, and that hardly any groups had even discussed the topic. The one exception seems to be the question of confidentiality, which appears to be taken for granted in most groups, although rarely discussed directly. This situation reminds me of something I learned about the efficiency experts who go into offices to try to improve system function. When they ask why something is done they way it is, the answer is always the same: "We've always done it that way." Individuals do better when they make conscious decisions. Systems also work better when they are consciously designed and adjusted.

In the modern world, we all have busy lives, and it can be hard to find several hours time (including travel) in the schedule for a group meeting, but once a month seems to me not often enough to maintain continuity, or to be available when something urgent comes up. I can see arguments on both sides for meeting in one place or for rotating. It would be more convenient to pick an office that was centrally located and make that the official meeting place. It might also feel more fair to have everyone share the responsibility, and have meetings rotate location.

The effects on the group of member absences can depend a lot on the size of the group. If there are only three people (as with some of our groups), then one absence can profoundly affect the members in attendance. But even in a larger group, absence can undermine the smooth functioning of the group. People who are away miss the presentation and continuity is compromised. The missing person's input is not available, and a solution may be overlooked. People can have strong reactions to others' absences, feeling abandoned and rejected, or unimportant, and these feelings may persist even when the absent member returns.

There are few reasons, outside of the purchase of snacks for the group, for there to be any money involved in most groups. The exceptions mentioned above are self-explanatory. I disagree that the cause of a group's dissolution lies in the lack of payment. It seems much more likely that other issues, and the failure to address them, are the cause.

If everyone is in agreement that they want to include reading and discussing books and articles, I think that can add a dimension to the work of the group that will enhance the case presentations and deepen the discussion. In many groups, members don't want anything that takes time away from case presentation itself.

Overall, I wish that all these topics were discussed by the group and that decisions were made consciously. Maybe a good time to do that would be whenever a new member joins the group. In the process if informing and assimilating the new person, all these issues could be reviewed.

In the next section, we will look at the main aspect of group functioning, the discussion of cases, problems, and issues. How clearly and consistently the structure is defined and maintained will determine, at least in part, how effectively these presentations are processed.

*Address*

*Structure*

# Chapter 6

# Presenting a Case

In this section we will examine the ways cases and issues are brought before the group, and the kinds of things that people need help with. We also look at how people feel about their presentations and about the feedback the group gives them.

Many groups have a prevailing perspective due to the members having trained together. Other groups have a diverse set of members, and see the variety of perspectives as an important asset. Containing feelings such as shame and anxiety is necessary if a presentation is going to be productive for the presenter and for the group.

## What kinds of issues do people present?

Many different kinds of issues are brought up and discussed in peer supervision group meetings. People mentioned situations of countertransference most often (twenty), including specifically feeling lost, stuck, frustrated, baffled, or angry at the patient (seventeen).

> Probably at this stage in what we're all struggling with, it's usually some issue with our own difficulties dealing with a patient. Although people don't necessarily say "I'm having this countertransference problem," that's usually what it turns out to be.
>
> [Female, 35 years practice, 15 years in PSG]

> It turns out usually to be a blind spot with the therapist presenting, that they're not connecting the dots in a certain way, or they're having a personal countertransference issue, or they think they're not getting it and actually they *are* getting it and doing just fine.
>
> [Female, 30 years practice, 30 years in PSG]

The group used to have a name: The Countertransference Group. We've strayed a bit from that focus, but it's still about personal upsets and dilemmas with patients. "I'm so angry at this person that I'm afraid I'm acting out." "I feel like I've made a terrible error," coming in with a sense of remorse or guilt. "I don't seem to be getting anywhere with this person." "What should I do with how much this patient is acting out?" "What am I missing here?"

[Male, 40 years practice, 15 years in PSG]

It's all about parataxical distortion—when the therapist takes on the feelings of the patient. This group has been very helpful when you have to differentiate that out.

[Female, 40 years practice, 18 years in PSG]

The more interesting stuff has to do with the dynamics, and trying to understand the psychodynamics of the patient, or the relationship between the therapist and the patient. So that if there's any blind spot the group can help them see it. And those cases seem to me to be the most fruitful discussions.

[Female, 25 years practice, 15 years in PSG]

It's mostly our countertransference issues, in the sense that we'll present a case that we're stuck on; we don't quite know what to do. Oftentimes, with me, I'll think the patient is in college when they're really in kindergarten. I'm expecting too much.

[Female, 35 years practice, 32 years in PSG]

Maybe you don't know that it's countertransference, and once you start discussing it you find out it is. When you know somebody for a long time you may understand what their issues are. We tend after all these years to keep having the same problems, and get hooked in the same places.

[Female, 35 years practice, 30 years in PSG]

Some people (ten) mentioned practice management issues, such as billing, cancellations, consultations, and ethical or legal questions.

Sometimes there are legal issues, things that frighten different members, when they get anxious about something.

[Female, 20 years practice, 12 years in PSG]

Sometimes it becomes clear that other clinicians need to be involved in the case, and that will get discussed. Sometimes one of us will pick up a portion of the case, to see a spouse or parent, and sometimes that's not a good idea.

[Female, 20 years practice, 15 years in PSG]

Some practice management issues, like insurance, unpaid bills, consultation with other therapists, and the like.

[Male, 30 years practice, 25 years in PSG]

An issue would be something that applies across the practice, like ending the session on time, or what to do when your practice hours drop down, or handling cancellations.

[Male, 10 years practice, 3 years in PSG]

Some people (eight) cited the stress of working with a suicidal or otherwise difficult patient.

Sometimes people will say, "I can't stand this case, I'm so frustrated." They need some clinical help to understand that their frustration is part of the diagnostic.

[Female, 20 years practice, 15 years in PSG]

We discuss difficult patients, in regard to group membership, as in "I brought a new patient into my group a few weeks ago, and now I'm wondering whether that was a disaster." I have a group in which people tend to subgroup into two levels of functioning and I'm trying to figure out how to manage that. I have a person who tends to monopolize, and I'm trying to work with that.

[Male, 15 years practice, 1 year in PSG]

The kinds of cases that usually get brought up are the more difficult patients, the ones who have attempted suicide, or talk more about suicide. Cases where a patient feels really stuck, they can't see any movement, even though they've been working with the therapist for a long time. Or a patient who's just difficult and the therapist finds himself really angry, or frustrated, and wants some feedback.

[Male, 10 years practice, 3 years in PSG]

Somebody has a patient that says "No, no, no, that's not it," to everything the therapist says, and we discuss how to help this patient move, how the therapist is going to modify a little bit to get some traction in the treatment.

[Female, 25 years practice, 1 year in PSG]

We're all pretty experienced therapists, so it's when someone feels that they're having trouble with a patient. Sometimes it's a crisis, a suicidal patient, or someone threatening to leave, and the therapist feeling that they don't know why, and wanting some support with it.

[Female, 25 years practice, 11 years in PSG]

For example, someone brought up a case of domestic abuse, where the wife got beaten fairly often by the father of her three kids. She wound up in the hospital twice. And she stays with him. The frustration of trying to work with her, the feeling of "What else can I do?"

[Male, 40 years practice, 7 years in PSG]

People often bring up situations where they're very concerned about the severity of a patient's acting out, such as the possibility of suicidality, acting out in some way that they'd like to get a handle on.

[Female, 40 years practice, 17 years in PSG]

Six people mentioned issues around money: setting, collecting, or raising fees, and how the current economy affects private practice.

Sometimes it's payment and insurance complications that create complications in the treatment relationship. We have had groups where we don't discuss a patient per se but we talk about how we are all feeling in the current financial situation, and how we might be feeling coming into the treatment.

[Female, 25 years practice, 1 year in PSG]

A few people (three) mentioned boundary issues, defining the therapeutic contract and space.

We discuss boundary issues, you might know this person. Sometimes we see other members of the family, and they might try to coordinate the treatment.

[Male, 16 years practice, 5 years in PSG]

Sometimes you're getting angry because the patient is jerking you around in terms of scheduling. Some of us are better than others at setting boundaries. Sometimes we talk about administrative issues that have nothing to do with a specific client.

[Female, 35 years practice, 30 years in PSG]

Some people (three) mentioned the question of how to manage patient termination, especially when the therapist thought it was premature.

Sometimes an unexpected termination can bring up a strong reaction. What's the best way to respond?

[Male, 10 years practice, 6 months in PSG]

We deal with anxiety that someone's not making enough progress with a patient, or anxiety that something's going on that's going to make the patient leave. The latter is probably the most frequent, that people are worried about losing the patient.

[Female, 40 years practice, 17 years in PSG]

Two people brought up the problem of therapist burnout. This is a common feeling for busy professionals.

We might discuss feeling in a professional funk, like you just hit the wall.

[Male, 10 years practice, 3 years in PSG]

We would often talk about your capacity for dealing with this difficult sort of patient, your aggression toward the patient, your feeling used up, or beat up. When you were feeling difficulties like that, that would be the priority.

[Female, 30 years practice, 3 years in PSG]

Two people mentioned their need to get a general review of a case, either an ongoing treatment or a brand-new patient.

Sometimes people feel like they have a very intense treatment going on and want some kind of review to get peer feedback about it.

[Female, 25 years practice, 11 years in PSG]

Sometimes people present a new patient—they just want to talk about someone they just started seeing and get some feedback.

[Male, 10 years practice, 3 years in PSG]

One person each mentioned these issues: therapist illness, diagnosis, working with dreams, managing medications, sharing new areas of study and learning, and practice marketing.

Somebody's always studying something new. So there's a fair amount of discussion of whatever one of us is into.

[Female, 20 years practice, 7 years in PSG]

One person had a strong reaction to some of the issues other group members brought up.

Some people will bring up very mundane things that they really should know. It's rather astounding. Sometimes it's a boundary issue. I'm surprised because the solution seems so basic, and obvious.

[Female, 25 years practice, 20 years in PSG]

Another person had a different take on the feelings toward the patient.

We discuss the question of "Do I really care about this person? I go
through the motions, I see them every week, but do I really care?"
Someone brought up something Freud had written that said what cures
people in therapy is love, and we discussed that for several meetings.

[Male, 40 years practice, 7 years in PSG]

## My own experience

All the topics mentioned in these responses have been discussed in my
group. Because all of us are psychoanalytically trained, we most often
address situations from the perspective of the therapist having some kind
of countertransferential reaction that interferes with clinical effectiveness.

Some other issues that we have discussed recently include suicidal
patients, medication advantages and drawbacks, dealing with insurance
companies and managed care, and how to best work with couples.

# What kinds of issues lead you to present a case?

This slightly different version of the previous question gets a little more
personal. Many people (sixteen) mentioned countertransference reactions, and personal feelings toward the patient they were not pleased to
have.

I remember presenting one patient who stimulated a lot of envy in me,
and competitive feelings, kept making me feel uncomfortably envious
of her life, even though she was the one coming to me for treatment.

[Female, 40 years practice, 15 years in PSG]

Sometimes I bring up someone because I can't stand them, and when
they're coming I feel nauseous.

[Female, 35 years practice, 30 years in PSG]

Often it's because I'm aware that the patient is making me angry, or
uncomfortable, in a way that I know has got to be countertransferential.
I know that I had better bring it up, because I'm going to get caught up
in something with this patient, and maybe say things that are not going
to be helpful.

[Female, 40 years practice, 17 years in PSG]

It's not often that something will make me angry, and I'm knowledgeable enough to know that it means something when I am. I don't often
say "I want to quit this case," but I have felt that way on occasion.

[Female, 20 years practice, 15 years in PSG]

I felt so pinned down by the patient that I completely lost my center of how to respond to her.

[Female, 35 years practice, 5 years in PSG]

I don't know how to intervene when they get angry at me, or what to say back when they're critical.

[Male, 10 years practice, 3 years in PSG]

I raise it if I'm so angry at this person that I'm afraid I'm acting out.

[Male, 40 years practice, 15 years in PSG]

Ten people said they brought up a case when they felt stuck, at an impasse, or unsure about how to proceed.

The feeling that I'm lost, that nothing's happening, that I don't know what I'm doing.

[Male, 30 years practice, 25 years in PSG]

When I find myself feeling, "I don't seem to be getting anywhere with this person."

[Male, 40 years practice, 15 years in PSG]

Nine people said they presented a patient when they believed they had made a mistake, or somehow mishandled the case.

I presented a case recently where I felt so unsuccessful, and I wanted to hear what other people would have done. Either to get validation that there was nothing else that could have been done, or some suggestions of what else I might have done.

[Female, 25 years practice, 8 years in PSG]

I feel like I've made a terrible error, coming in with a sense of remorse or guilt.

[Male, 40 years practice, 15 years in PSG]

Eight people said they brought up difficult or challenging patients.

I've also talked about people who are hard to engage fully in the process, where there's a more prolonged period where it's hard to get that traction, and how to consider altering my style.

[Female, 25 years practice, 1 year in PSG]

I often brought up the problems of managing highly suicidal patients and whether they needed to be in the hospital. We try to minimize hospitalizations, and you really need the group support sometimes to make that call. I would have difficulty with certain kinds of interventions, like irreverence, or sense of humor, and colleagues would share how they would handle the situation and would get very specific. They use a lot of metaphors. They would help me get to a better metaphor.

[Female, 30 years practice, 3 years in PSG]

I'll present something when I'm feeling at a loss. Recently I've been struggling with a very depressed patient and I can't seem to do anything. She's on medications of all varieties, had shock treatment, a real serious depression. And it's kind of reassuring to hear that other people don't like those kinds of cases either.

[Female, 20 years practice, 7 years in PSG]

Six people said they asked for help when they felt they didn't know enough about a particular topic or issue, and wanted to draw on the expertise of the group.

If clients came in around a certain theme that I felt I didn't have a lot of experience with or felt challenged by clinically, I would bring that up.

[Female, 5 years practice, 1 year in PSG]

Sometimes it's just panic, like when I had a case of multiple personality, and I would have gone crazy if the group didn't help me. That was not countertransference, that was just not knowing how to handle something.

[Female, 45 years practice, 30 years in PSG]

Six people said they were prompted to discuss a case when they had the impression that they were somehow missing something.

There's something I'm missing and I want the group to maybe hear it for me. I need to get a little feedback about what other people hear. Sometimes if I'm not understanding what a patient has told me, if they're giving me a message and I feel like I don't get the message, so I want feedback from others about that.

[Female, 25 years practice, 15 years in PSG]

I bring it up when someone really has me puzzled, and I feel I'm not doing as good a job as I would like to do, when I'm not doing the work I want to do, or going as deeply as I think I might be able to because I'm missing something to have the capacity to do so.

[Female, 30 years practice, 30 years in PSG]

I talk about where I feel my own shame of not helping enough or understanding enough. Am I missing something? Am I having blind spots with a patient?

[Male, 15 years practice, 5 years in PSG]

Generally I'll have this feeling in the pit of my stomach, that I'm just not helping someone with their issue, and I don't know why. I'll feel kind of stuck and helpless, and like my interpretations are off-base or being rejected in some way.
[Female, 20 years practice, 12 years in PSG]

I see a new patient and it seems like we have a good session, and I think he's going to call and make another appointment, but he never calls. And then I find out that he called the second name on the list of referrals, and I was really surprised, and wanted some feedback as to what might have happened, because I usually read things very clearly.
[Female, 35 years practice, 30 years in PSG]

With one patient, I was having difficulty understanding what was going on. The group was very helpful, partly because everybody in the group felt so differently about this patient than I did. It was as though I had a block in seeing something about her. The whole group had a reaction to this patient that I didn't have. It made me think that I was missing something about that patient. It made me go back and listen a little differently.
[Female, 35 years practice, 15 years in PSG]

Three people mentioned the question of patient termination.

One time it was about a termination that I felt didn't go that well, even though the patient had been in treatment three or four years, there was something abrupt and unresolved about it, and I wanted to process that.
[Female, 25 years practice, 1 year in PSG]

I brought up someone who wanted to leave therapy. I didn't have an issue with it, I thought it was a good time for him to leave therapy, but I was second-guessing myself and I wanted to make sure that there wasn't something else I should do to help him reconsider before he left.
[Male, 10 years practice, 3 years in PSG]

One person each mentioned these issues: referrals, marketing, practice management, and one said they might bring up a case simply because it might be interesting for the group to discuss.

Sometimes it's because a patient is particularly interesting, and probably going to be complicated, and I want to bring it up early so people know who it is when I talk about them later. I've done that several times.
[Female, 40 years practice, 17 years in PSG]

A few people mentioned some very specific situations they had raised over the years.

> An example is what I'll present in the next meeting, which is one of my favorite groups, a really rich, dynamic, interpersonally juicy group with a lot of integrity. I've brought in three new members in the last few months. One of them left very abruptly. One of them I think I need to ask to leave, because I think he's really toxic to the group. I haven't done that in many years. I want to work through the question of wheth er that's an appropriate thing to do, or am I acting something out egregiously. Is it too late? Has the group already been damaged? I think it has been in some ways. Two other members have started talking about leaving, and I think it's related to this guy's presence, and nobody's naming that. He hasn't been around long enough, and he's explicitly not willing to do interpersonal work, which I did not know when I brought him in. He pulled the wool over my eyes. So it's a really messy, ugly, awful situation, and I'm really glad we're meeting tomorrow, because I really need to get some help with it.
>
> [Male, 15 years practice, 1 year in PSG]

> I once presented a situation in which a patient wrote me a letter in which he said he was going to get a gun and shoot someone. I hadn't seen the patient in over a month and, while I was pretty sure that it was a fantasy, I couldn't be absolutely certain. The law is very clear on this issue that we have a "duty to warn," even though I wasn't sure who I was warning. The group unanimously agreed that I had to call the police. So I did, very reluctantly, and they picked him up and hospitalized him over a weekend. He was very traumatized by the incident, felt very betrayed by me, and quit treatment for several years, although he did ultimately return to seeing me. It's one of the few things I regret in my clinical work over thirty years. I wish I hadn't done it. I wish I had trusted my clinical judgment, and not turned the responsibility for the decision over to the group.
>
> [Male, 30 years practice, 25 years in PSG]

> Once I talked about a patient who was beautiful, a model, and she turned out to be a man, and the group went crazy talking about my fantasies.
>
> [Male, 40 years practice, 7 years in PSG]

## My own experience

When I have an issue to present, it's usually about feeling stuck. The patient isn't moving, and I'm wondering what I'm missing. I don't have this feeling very often, so I know there's something that needs looking at. Sometimes I simply feel baffled—what the hell is *that*? Again, not a normal response for me. I often like to discuss a new patient, not because there's any particular problem, but just to get an overview, some sense of where we're heading in the treatment and what to watch out for.

Anything that feels out of the ordinary is something that could potentially point to a problem that needs looking at. Paying attention to those little hints that something is not normal as soon as they arise can save a lot of difficulty later on.

## How often do you present a case?

People vary greatly in how often they use the group to discuss a case. Most people (fifteen) said they present only once or twice out of ten meetings; seven people said they present three or four times out of ten; three people said they present five or six times; two people said they present seven or eight times out of ten meetings; and seven people said they present at almost every meeting.

Some groups have an agreement that they divide the time so that everyone gets to present.

> We usually all present something, more often than not.
> [Female, 35 years practice, 30 years in PSG]

Several people mentioned that they are actively engaged even when someone else is presenting.

> I often add something to someone else's presentation. I often don't realize I've got an issue that's bothering me until someone else presents that issue and it bubbles up.
> [Female, 20 years practice, 12 years in PSG]

> I present maybe two out of ten meetings. But in a way that dovetails or adds to what someone else presents, then I present every time.
> [Male, 15 years practice, 1 year in PSG]

People are conscious of how much group time they are taking.

> I'm pretty good about speaking up. But I worry about speaking too much. I worry that I'm participating too much rather than too little.
> [Female, 20 years practice, 12 years in PSG]

A few people linked the frequency of presentation to other factors.

> For me it depends a lot on what's going on in my life outside the group, whether I'm distracted by personal things, and sometimes I just don't

have that kind of energy. But when I'm feeling free of things in my private life I will present a little more frequently.

[Female, 25 years practice, 15 years in PSG]

It totally depends on what's going on. I could present for three or four times, and then not for a couple of months.

[Female, 25 years practice, 15 years in PSG]

**My own experience**

I don't present very often, maybe once or twice out of ten meetings, because I find that I don't feel stuck or lost very often. I still get a lot from the group, even when I'm not presenting, because I learn so much from the discussions around other people's presentations.

# Are you ever nervous about presenting a case?

Most people have some anxiety about revealing how they work. Twenty-four people said they felt nervous about presenting a case and revealing themselves; ten said they were not, particularly in their peer supervision group, where they felt safe enough to disclose their weaknesses.

Several people contrasted their peer group with the groups they had been in during training.

I had had the background of presenting in analytic training, where people could be so hostile and competitive, and there was a group leader who just fed on that. It was horrible. He seemed to pit us against each other for some reason, like sport. Coming out of that, I was a little reluctant to join a group, and I have found this group to be extremely supportive, and I'm not nervous. I love that when I need help I can get it. People are really good to each other.

[Female, 20 years practice, 12 years in PSG]

I have rarely had good supervision in my training. I've had some, and that's been absolutely delicious, but mostly it's not been very helpful. So I tend to want to present something that I already understand, and I'm working to be able to present things I need help with.

[Male, 15 years practice, 1 year in PSG]

The cases that get brought up are the most difficult and challenging; otherwise they wouldn't be causing problems for the therapist. Nevertheless, revealing mistakes can induce feelings of shame.

The group is quite good about people sharing that anxiety. They'll say, "I feel a lot of shame about this." The cases I present are the ones where I'm having the most trouble and I don't feel like I know what's going on. There are times where I feel so incompetent, or I've done something that's such a blunder, that it's embarrassing to reveal.

[Female, 25 years practice, 11 years in PSG]

There's always a little anxiety. It has to do with issues of embarrassment and shame.

[Male, 45 years practice, 20 years in PSG]

I'm revealing that I don't know enough that I *should* know. It shows my vulnerability, that somehow I'm not doing a good job with a patient.

[Female, 30 years practice, 8 months in PSG]

If I think I've done something really stupid or wrong, I'll be a little nervous. The group isn't shaming, but I still find it a little embarrassing.

[Male, 30 years practice, 25 years in PSG]

I might be a little anxious about embarrassing myself. I don't want to let people see how incompetent I am. I don't want to show how stupid I can be, or how ignorant I am. Will I be judged? Is this a harshly critical group, or a supportive and empathic group? When I present I'm much harder on myself than they are on me. I have to soothe my own internal critic first and then I can present.

[Male, 15 years practice, 5 years in PSG]

When we're nervous that gets talked about. It comes from some sense that some incompetence will be exposed. How could I be a respected practitioner when I'm fucking up with this case?

[Male, 40 years practice, 15 years in PSG]

People can worry about how others see them, especially when they know that they haven't done their best work, and can expect some critical feedback.

I say, "Let me tell you what I did"—I anticipate the group's going to judge me even though I know they won't.

[Female, 35 years practice, 2 years in PSG]

Occasionally I'm nervous, if I feel clueless, if I'm not on top of it, if I'm inept. If I have a little bit of a handle on what's happening, I'm fine. But it wouldn't keep me from presenting. It might motivate the presentation because I would feel I need help with this.

[Female, 25 years practice, 15 years in PSG]

Sometimes people *expect* to be criticized for their working style.

> One of my colleagues is kind of a hard-liner analyst, and will take very strong analytic positions I don't necessarily buy. So I'm sometimes prepared for that.
>
> [Female, 20 years practice, 7 years in PSG]

> Many of the people have a lot of experience, and at times my nervousness is because my more liberal interpretation of what psychoanalysis is might not match what *they* think it is. Some of them tend to be a little more rigid.
>
> [Male, 40 years practice, 7 years in PSG]

Because peer groups are often a source of referrals, members want to look their best. At times, other group members' judgments can have consequences.

> I'm sure I was nervous, because of the exposure. If you're going to talk about cases that you really need help with, you're going to be exposing where you're inadequate. There was always this tension between wanting to get the help and to use the group, wanting to bring myself in, and wanting my peers to think well of me.
>
> [Female, 40 years practice, 15 years in PSG]

> The anxiety would be about appearing incompetent, looking as if you're struggling with something others wouldn't struggle with. There's always that hope of being someone people would make referrals to, and if you're looking like someone who can't seem to handle a case that doesn't seem that difficult, then I may be worried that they're thinking, "Gosh, I won't refer to him."
>
> [Male, 10 years practice, 3 years in PSG]

It was often a relief to be able to admit to the anxiety.

> I'm able to say, "I really screwed up. Wait till you hear this. This is something I'll never publish in the journals."
>
> [Female, 35 years practice, 32 years in PSG]

> There have been occasions where I was nervous. Probably feeling that I should know more about a certain subject than I do. The good thing is that it can be talked about, and we've all taken turns from time to time saying, "I'm actually nervous talking about this." Maybe not until the discussion is complete do we realize that our awkwardness in discussing it was understandable and okay.
>
> [Female, 20 years practice, 15 years in PSG]

Some people said that their "nerves" were more a feeling of excitement or urgency.

> My only concern is I don't feel organized enough in making a presentation.
>
> [Female, 10 years practice, 6 years in PSG]

> The concern is to be concise, and I often have some apprehension about being concise and clear in the allotted amount of time, making sure that I'm focusing on the issue that I need assistance with.
>
> [Female, 25 years practice, 8 years in PSG]

> I sometimes feel a lot of urgency about whatever I'm presenting.
>
> [Female, 35 years practice, 30 years in PSG]

> I'm always nervous about presenting a case. Part of it is not knowing that I'm going to be clear enough. I don't take much in the way of notes, and whenever I'm presenting a case I'm always worried if I'm going to get to the point where I'm clear about what I want, or am I just going to ramble. I don't think my anxiety is about people's responses, because I feel at this point that we're very kind to each other, for the most part. There's not a feeling of danger in the group.
>
> [Female, 40 years practice, 17 years in PSG]

> Am I getting all the information I need to have gotten in order to present this well? Am I describing it well? I never prepare for it, I just trust that what is important will come out and I will get my point across and people will understand what this case is about and how I've participated in it.
>
> [Female, 30 years practice, 30 years in PSG]

The people who said they did not feel nervous about presenting usually attributed their comfort in revealing themselves to their trust in the group.

> I've known these people a long time; they know me, warts and all. And I'm able to be embarrassed, able to be foolish.
>
> [Female, 35 years practice, 30 years in PSG]

> I feel very supported there. It's very safe that you can bring things where you're not doing your best and get a lot of empathy.
>
> [Female, 35 years practice, 5 years in PSG]

## My own experience

I am rarely nervous about presenting a case, because I know group is a safe place and I won't be shamed for my behavior. I don't always like having to reveal that I don't know what's going on, but I do it because I know I'll feel better afterward and get the help I need. We are a very supportive group, and have created a safe space for everyone.

# Was there ever a case you didn't bring up because of concern about the group's reaction?

Sometimes we know that we've done or said something questionable. If we don't discuss that with the group we could miss an opportunity for real discovery: What could have led me to do that?

Only two people said that they might have censored themselves and avoided talking about a case they needed help with because they were worried about what the group might say. Neither could remember the details of the situation and what might have dissuaded them from bringing it up. But others admitted that there were some situations they might have kept silent about.

> It's always a boundary issue, where I'm going to stretch a boundary a little bit. I have the sense that there was something that I kept silencing myself about.
>
> [Female, 20 years practice, 7 years in PSG]

> I tend to be pretty forthcoming, but there might be issues that I wouldn't bring up, process issues in the group, that I wouldn't bring up because of anxiety.
>
> [Female, 35 years practice, 2 years in PSG]

> There were some interventions I didn't bring up because I wondered about the boundaries.
>
> [Female, 30 years practice, 3 years in PSG]

> I don't think that there are any situations where I've thought, "Oh, I couldn't let them know about that, they wouldn't think well of me." There are moments in the group processing that have been a little difficult, when I've been hesitant to speak to something directly, and have sat and silently tried to figure out. I was upset when I felt that I wasn't being heard, or didn't get what I needed, or when people in the group are missing the point and it's frustrating and annoying, and how to work with that. It doesn't mean I don't do it, but I'm aware that this could be hard for me.
>
> [Male, 15 years practice, 1 year in PSG]

A few people said they had avoided discussing a case, but not out of fear of what the group might say.

> I didn't bring up a case where they all knew the patient .
>                        [Female, 25 years practice, 8 years in PSG]

Several people said that they had the feeling, but didn't give in to the impulse to withhold.

> I know there have been times where I've felt like not bringing it up, but then I have and been glad that I did.
>                        [Female, 25 years practice, 11 years in PSG]

> I've had cases where I was concerned about the reaction, but never to the extent that I wouldn't bring it up if I needed help with it.
>                        [Female, 25 years practice, 15 years in PSG]

### My own experience
If I ever avoided bringing up a case that I needed to discuss, it could only have been many years ago, when I first joined the group and didn't feel safe with them yet. I don't have any conscious memory of doing it, but I couldn't swear that it never happened. I don't think it would happen now, because I would be able to start by addressing the fear about bringing up the case. That fear, in and of itself, would probably say something important about the patient and about the impasse.

## How do you process the feedback you get?

A person presents a case, and the group gives feedback, asks questions, and makes suggestions. I asked people to explain how they use what they get from the group.

People are often very clear about what kind of feedback they want, in terms of form and content.

> I use the feedback I get in the group to adjust my focus or style with a patient. If the feedback makes good sense to me, I try to incorporate it into my approach with the patient. You get different angles and perspectives on what's going on, maybe a dynamic of the patient or the process that you hadn't fully appreciated, or even seen, or recognized the importance of—something you overlooked or underestimated.
>                         [Female, 25 years practice, 1 year in PSG]

Unless there's someone that I really am struggling with, that I want
feedback and support with, I don't go there looking for advice.
[Male, 15 years practice, 5 years in PSG]

I see things differently. I get freed up from whatever was tying me up. I
identify what was tying me up. The most important thing is getting the
right emotional communications from your fellow members.
[Female, 35 years practice, 5 years in PSG]

Having to articulate and explain your own thinking about a case is itself
useful, separate from any feedback the group may give.

One of the things that happens with me is that as I present an issue, and
as people start to ask questions, I'll get a lot clearer. So it looks like as
if I'm not really receiving help, and yet it's been enormously helpful.
Because the people in the group think so much like I think, I start to get
what they're going to ask even before they begin to talk.
[Male, 15 years practice, 1 year in PSG]

Their impact on each other would be part of a process, and would resonate in various ways with what was going on in me. There was a very
clear understanding that there was no right or wrong, so a consensus
was never required. But it helped you to articulate why your ideas were
different.
[Female, 30 years practice, 3 years in PSG]

Many people said that they got a lot of insight and information when
others were presenting cases.

I get as much working and listening to another case as I do working on
my own case.
[Female, 25 years practice, 1 year in PSG]

Even when I'm not presenting there's a lot that I'm taking in. I feel
energized and redirected with some patients based on some things that
were said there.
[Male, 10 years practice, 3 years in PSG]

A few people said they took notes about what other group members offered.

I just try to absorb the feedback. I sometimes take notes during the
group, but I seldom look at them afterwards. I more prefer to just let it
filter through me, especially since it's mostly countertransference. I
want it to help shift something inside of me so I feel freer or better un-

derstand what's going on with me. So I don't do much structurally with it.

[Female, 25 years practice, 11 years in PSG]

Sometimes I'll take notes on what's being said. Sometimes we'll mirror what's being said as a way of making sure that we really understood what the person was saying.

[Female, 25 years practice, 8 years in PSG]

I'm a real note taker, so if I hear something that strikes a chord with me I write it down and put it in the case file. And then, when it's time to see the patient again, I take a few minutes to look at it and think about how it might affect what I say in the session.

[Female, 10 years practice, 6 years in PSG]

Sometimes I write notes after the group, of things that helped me and I don't want to forget. I take it very seriously, and it really expands my work with the client when I go back to the office. It refocuses me, and gives me a kind of confidence. Very often I feel like I'm not so off-base as I thought I was before.

[Female, 20 years practice, 12 years in PSG]

I'm the only one in any of the groups I've been in who writes down notes during the feedback. Because I'm so affectively involved in the presentation, and I'm concerned that I won't hear what people are telling me, I will write as best I can some of the things that people are saying to me. Sometimes it could be a question that got me thinking about something that I hadn't thought about.

[Female, 35 years practice, 2 years in PSG]

Many people said they edit as they go along, sifting through what is offered.

Sometimes I'm eliminating it as it's coming at me, and I'm thinking, "Oh, that's a really bad idea." I'm sifting through it as it happens. Or I might say to myself, "Oh, that's a really good idea. I'll have to remember that."

[Male, 10 years practice, 3 years in PSG]

You get all kinds of reactions, and you take hold of the ones you can use.

[Female, 45 years practice, 30 years in PSG]

I think about it, I consider it. I think either "There's some validity to that," or "There's absolutely no validity to that." I might throw it back to the group and ask what made them go in that particular direction. I might say, "I don't agree with you," or maybe "No, that's not what's really going on."

[Female, 25 years practice, 20 years in PSG]

I often try to think about it, to understand, to accept it, and other times I don't accept it because I think that they were missing something important.

[Male, 40 years practice, 7 years in PSG]

Most people said they just listened, tried to take in what was being offered, and thought about it afterward.

I listen pretty carefully, and I look for where my personality might be coming into the situation, whatever character piece is mine. It gives me a chance to identify that piece.

[Female, 35 years practice, 30 years in PSG]

I think about what the members tell me and use the suggestions if I think they are applicable. Sometimes members disagree about aspects of a case. The most helpful comments are usually about my own reactions to the patient and that helps to further my understanding of my countertransference and therefore helps me to use it.

[Female, 35 years practice, 15 years in PSG]

Both the feedback and the participation in the group, even when it's not explicitly about my cases, are useful, because that makes me think about my groups, and do I want to talk about that. It makes me think about how I manage a situation compared to how other people manage it. It adds a layer of reflection that I might not do otherwise because I'm busy doing the work. So it creates a space in my own mind, certainly in the group. But also between meetings I'm aware that I'm thinking about things a little more.

[Male, 15 years practice, 1 year in PSG]

I listen very intently to the feedback. I respect all of them, and I find that their comments are usually very helpful. They're very different and they all have different takes.

[Female, 20 years practice, 7 years in PSG]

Some people said they accept and reject advice as the group proceeds.

I just ignore the ones adding to the confusion and go with the ones that resonate with me and my patient.

[Male, 10 years practice, 3 years in PSG]

It's not really confusing, because I can figure out what's on target. In the group session I already know what I won't use.

[Female, 40 years practice, 18 years in PSG]

It's not confusing because I reject what doesn't feel right.

[Male, 30 years practice, 25 years in PSG]

It's not confusing because I'm going to take what fits for me and leave the rest.

[Male, 15 years practice, 1 year in PSG]

This person said she tried not to think about the feedback.

I walk out of the group and I don't think about all the input. I get into the session, and then it flows. Ninety-nine percent of the time there's a change. It's fantastic.

[Female, 40 years practice, 18 years in PSG]

In some ways, the effects of presenting a case in peer group are mysterious.

In some magic way, when you go back to your patient after the group has given feedback, you work better with the patient.

[Female, 45 years practice, 30 years in PSG]

As people talk, I sift out the suggestions that don't resonate with me. I hold on to the other suggestions and have a few days before I see the patient again to let the material percolate. When I see the patient again I find that I'm taking a different tack and the stuck feeling disappears.

[Male, 30 years practice, 25 years in PSG]

I listen carefully, and I sit with it. I let it percolate. Do I agree with them? Don't I agree with them? Then I come back to the office and I listen to the patient and I resonate with what was discussed in the peer group. Then I have the option of integrating it with the work, or not.

[Male, 15 years practice, 5 years in PSG]

It immediately affects the way I hear and think about the person in the next session. There's an immediate carryover. I may even speak differently to the person who's been discussed, which is astounding to me, that it has that big an impact.

[Female, 25 years practice, 15 years in PSG]

Sometimes someone will make an interpretation about my case that will totally open up an area I wasn't even looking at, and moves the therapy in leaps and bounds.

[Female, 25 years practice, 15 years in PSG]

Some people said that being in a long-term group with others who know them well was a tremendous help.

> I find feedback is useful mainly to try to grab hold of something getting in our way in working with a patient. We're all senior enough to know how to work with patients. Our stuckness is generally our own stuff coming up in some kind of manner, and being with people who know us pretty well over time is helpful in getting to this stuff pretty quickly. I have found discussing things in the group has also at times helped me to deal with what I felt was an overreaction on my part, and the group could be a leveling influence with our own self-expectations, and has been with me.
>
>                       [Female, 40 years practice, 17 years in PSG]

> Some of the most dramatic, gripping, and greatly valued moments occur because the group knows what's going on in my life and can make the connection. Of course I've thought about it but I haven't really understood it.
>
>                       [Male, 40 years practice, 15 years in PSG]

> Unless I specifically ask for advice or suggestions, I'm much more interested in being heard and understood, in being felt. I know that my problem-solving process is a good one, and what usually ignites it is to get something off my chest, and from there I can take that experience of being heard and understood and find my way.
>
>                       [Male, 10 years practice, 6 months in PSG]

This person mentioned a specific issue the group had helped her with.

> The group is really helpful in making me understand that I'm expecting too much, and that's my issue.
>
>                       [Female, 35 years practice, 30 years in PSG]

One person cited a specific example of how the group had been useful.

> Someone in the group said about a case of mine, because she sees the sibling, to be more confrontational with a single mother who was missing sessions because she was so disorganized. And I was, but I don't think I handled it well. And then six months later, I was bringing up something about the patient and my colleague said that she had the impression, through the sibling she sees, that the patient was disorganized before she was a mother. That helped me because the following week I was more able to confront her and my boundaries were firmer.
>
>                       [Female, 35 years practice, 32 years in PSG]

## My own experience

I find that presenting a case to the group works best when I simply listen to what the group has to say, try not to judge what they're saying, don't think too hard about it, let it simmer and percolate, and see what comes to mind when next working with the patient. There is a conscious process, of rationally weighing the feedback and seeing how it applies, and also an unconscious process, in which things resonate and reverberate somewhere deep, and both combine to shift my perspective and my responses when I'm in the room with that patient.

# How useful is the feedback?

It seems obvious that there will be occasions when the group is not helpful, gives advice that turns out not so well, or is stumped. Yet twelve people said that presenting in their peer group was always useful.

> It varies from very useful to less useful, but never not useful.
> [Female, 25 years practice, 8 years in PSG]

If the group is large enough, with enough different points of view, the odds that no one will find a way to be helpful are minimized.

> Some of what people say I immediately reject as unhelpful. But there are a lot of people in the group and something is always useful.
> [Male, 30 years practice, 25 years in PSG]

> What's become so good about the group is that we all have different backgrounds. So there'll be some very different ways of conceptualizing what's going on. Then there'll be an argument in front of me about what I've presented. And I might say, "I'm not fully understanding that, help me understand that," or "I'm still having trouble accepting that," or that kind of thing.
> [Male, 40 years practice, 15 years in PSG]

People gave different explanations for the feedback failing to help.

> In another peer group the feedback was often dogmatic and rigid: "There's an alcohol problem and you must send this person to AA." You couldn't talk past that, because it's so adamant, that's the rule. That was very unhelpful.
> [Female, 25 years practice, 15 years in PSG]

It's not useful when it seems too simplistic, something I've tried and it didn't work, or I just can't imagine trying it. Or it's way too psychoana-lytically elaborate, it seems too convoluted to me.

[Male, 10 years practice, 3 years in PSG]

Sometimes people are on kicks. They've gone to a workshop or they're studying something that's not yet comfortably integrated into my way of working. I listen, and I consider it, but it may not be very helpful to me because of my style.

[Female, 20 years practice, 12 years in PSG]

Sometimes people will want to give help more than I want to get it. They'll keep going after I've gotten what I needed, and I have to say, "I've got it, no more." Or people will get triggered, and go off in a di-rection that has nothing to do with my problem.

[Female, 25 years practice, 15 years in PSG]

It's not useful when they tell me things I've already tried.

[Female, 20 years practice, 7 years in PSG]

It's not possible for the others to know the patient as well as I do.

[Female, 35 years practice, 32 years in PSG]

I didn't find it so helpful if they told me what I ought to do, because stylistically we were all pretty different.

[Female, 40 years practice, 15 years in PSG]

Sometimes it's not applicable to how you're thinking about a case.

[Female, 10 years practice, 6 years in PSG]

When I get feedback of the sort of, "You should do this," I tend to balk a little bit. That may just be my personality.

[Male, 10 years practice, 6 months in PSG]

There are times I can incorporate it more easily than others. There are times when what people are saying may be true, but it isn't what I'm working on, or what I'm doing, it's off on a tangent.

[Female, 40 years practice, 17 years in PSG]

Some people said that, if the feedback was not helpful, they would ex-press their reactions.

If the feedback isn't useful I say so. I would say, "We're going in the wrong direction," or I would try to refocus what I need. Sometimes the feedback isn't quite what I'm asking but it can still be useful. If it isn't

useful I wouldn't just pretend that it is. I would speak to that, if it happened.

> [Female, 35 years practice, 2 years in PSG]

It can sometimes take a while for the usefulness to emerge.

> I may not feel the usefulness of everything the group is telling me in
> the meeting, or even right after, but then when I'm with the patient
> again I really feel the help.
>
> [Female, 40 years practice, 17 years in PSG]

Some people cited specific examples.

> There was one time recently where I thought that everyone was react-
> ing too personally, rather than clinically. What happened with the case
> was almost opposite to what people were saying. Sometimes people
> bring in opinions that aren't really clinical. It's just their own anxiety. I
> found that session extremely unhelpful.
>
> [Female, 35 years practice, 30 years in PSG]

> There was one patient a number of years ago where it wasn't useful.
> They were feeling so frustrated with the patient that they couldn't be
> useful, and I ended up going for supervision.
>
> [Female, 35 years practice, 15 years in PSG]

> All the groups I do are with gay men, and I remember a time when I
> felt like I was having to teach Gay 101 for one of the other people who
> didn't get something, and that was not the issue that we were talking
> about. But I had to educate them and get past that, and I was wondering
> if it was even worth doing that. It was interesting to have that experi-
> ence again, because it's an experience I have had many times, and it's
> an experience that my group members have all the time.
>
> [Male, 15 years practice, 1 year in PSG]

## My own experience
In my own group, there are so many people giving feedback that it's very
likely that at least one person will say something that doesn't help me.
But often when many people give different opinions, even though some
comments may seem to contradict others, it's all helpful. Almost every
comment or question illuminates something, or reorganizes my thinking
in some way.

# Is the feedback ever confusing?

When the group is in agreement about what to do, it's easy to follow the advice. But what happens when there is no consensus? Nine people said it was sometimes confusing.

> Early in my career I used to find the feedback flooding and overstimulating, and getting all the different ideas was overwhelming. That happens much less now, because I'm much more confident. I still worry about letting go of my own voice and following someone else's advice. That was more true when I had supervisors and I would idealize them and lose my own instincts. There's always that feeling I'm having of not wanting to do exactly what someone's telling me to do.
>
> [Female, 25 years practice, 11 years in PSG]

> Sometimes it can be overload. In a group with a moderator we look to him or her, but when it's peer supervision at times it could get a bit daunting, and I found it hard to process.
>
> [Female, 5 years practice, 1 year in PSG]

> Sometimes it is confusing, and what I tend to do is call people between meetings to ask their opinion.
>
> [Female, 30 years practice, 8 months in PSG

Four other people said that, while it might at times be confusing, they didn't regard the confusion as a negative state to be in.

> There can be pursued discussion about that, stylistic differences, and so on. Sometimes it leaves me wondering about my own way of working. I think it makes me question myself, but in a useful way.
>
> [Female, 25 years practice, 1 year in PSG]

> I'm comfortable sitting with not knowing. I have an hour train ride back home to sit with it and process it.
>
> [Male, 15 years practice, 5 years in PSG]

> It did sometimes feel confusing, but I kind of liked it, because it felt like stirring stuff up, and I didn't mind that confusion.
>
> [Female, 40 years practice, 15 years in PSG]

> I think confusion is a good thing. It's how you get from A to B. So if I'm confused I don't see that as a negative. I'll say I'm confused, and we'll talk about it, and usually it ends up in a good place.
>
> [Female, 20 years practice, 15 years in PSG]

Twenty-one people said it was not confusing, and that they liked having so many divergent opinions.

> It's not confusing. I like that there's different ways of looking at everything.
>
> [Female, 35 years practice, 30 years in PSG]

> That kind of dialogue, at least for me, opens up the field a little bit, so that I can walk away from it with a feeling of freedom. Sometimes I won't even think of it until the next session with the patient, and I'll suddenly think of something someone said in group, maybe something to say that someone suggested, and it may not be something I would have thought of on my own.
>
> [Female, 40 years practice, 17 years in PSG]

> It's a pretty cohesive group, but even when they have different opinions it becomes exciting to look at them, not confusing. I can really be stimulated by the differences.
>
> [Female, 25 years practice, 8 years in PSG]

Another portion of those who found it not confusing said that the group usually reached a consensus.

> The group may throw out a lot of opinions, and may feel like it's not forming anything, but generally there's a coalescing into some integrated way before the end. It doesn't stay fragmented. It generally comes together in some helpful way.
>
> [Female, 20 years practice, 12 years in PSG]

**My own experience**

Personally I don't mind a little confusion—it's a sign that some learning is taking place and that things are being reorganized. I already had some confusion when I came to group—that's why I'm presenting the case. So I think it's useful to try to tolerate the discomfort of a temporary confusion.

Of course, if the confusion persists, even after meeting with the patient again, then more discussion is required. I find that this hardly ever happens.

# How do you use the parallel process in the group when a case is being presented?

How this question is answered seems to hinge on how many of the group members are group therapists, and are familiar and at ease with group process. Only one person said they did not ever notice parallel process in a case presentation. In most instances, what occurs is that feelings that the patient evokes in the therapist are evoked in the group during the presentation. Understanding what the feelings are, and how they get brought out, can shed light on the dynamics of the patient and on the relationship between the patient and the therapist.

Normally one of the group members will call the group's attention to what they have observed.

> Someone who might be seeing it would step in and point out that it's happening.
>> [Female, 25 years practice, 8 years in PSG]

> One of the members is a specialist in groups, and he'll point it out. Then we move into the territory of our own group process. It's just additional useful information.
>> [Male, 40 years practice, 15 years in PSG]

> If the group is in a flurry of anxiety, someone might say that this seems to be what's going on in the therapy. That usually stops whatever the emotional reaction is that's being played out in the group. It usually interferes with it. Once it's raised to a conscious level it stops.
>> [Female, 25 years practice, 15 years in PSG]

> Sometimes there's a vociferous disagreement about it, and we'll realize that it relates to something that's going on with the patient.
>> [Female, 25 years practice, 11 years in PSG]

> Usually we all see it, and someone will very gently point it out. It's part of the whole point of being in supervision, of being blind to our own countertransference, so it's useful. It illuminates some aspect of the case.
>> [Female, 20 years practice, 7 years in PSG]

Some people were able to describe the phenomenon very clearly, and the energy that can come with it.

> Hopefully I or one of the other members will say, "It occurs to me that right here and now is somehow reflective of the dilemma that you're describing in your group as well." Somebody will notice and speak to it. I might sit with it for a little while, because you don't want to interrupt the person who's talking about how confusing their patient is, but when I experience them as confusing and usually they're pretty intelligible, I might say, "I'm having this experience, I wonder if it's connected. Is there a way we can use this?" It can help the person under-

stand something that's going on for them in their group. But if it's larger than just how they're presenting, like if we're all giving the person advice, and that's what happens in their group, and they're asking how do they get the group not to give advice to each other, I might identify that, and then we might laugh. Here we are doing the very same thing. And then we would try to understand how that happened.

[Female, 35 years practice, 2 years in PSG]

We all listen for parallel process as informative of what the process might be with a patient, and what the transference is, what the countertransference is, but for me it's what keeps this group interesting. I'm not interested in sitting with colleagues and talking about theory. I'm bored to tears. It brings it alive for me if I'm living it.

[Male, 15 years practice, 1 year in PSG]

Some groups are open to looking at the phenomenon, and some are not.

If I'm expressing anxiety about a case I notice some members are zoning out. I rarely point it out. I'm one of the few people who are likely to say that a presentation is inducing feelings in me.

[Female, 25 years practice, 20 years in PSG]

We would try to use it. But when we were all in it, it was hard to step back and analyze it. I don't think it was a particularly useful.

[Female, 40 years practice, 15 years in PSG]

I try to point it out, and sometimes they're open to hearing it and experiencing it, and sometimes they aren't.

[Male, 15 years practice, 5 years in PSG]

Several people remembered specific examples of parallel process.

I find that sometimes a lot of people will be talking at once, and talking over each other and not listening, and generally the group is aware enough to stop and say, "Hey, what's going on with this case that we're doing that?" And almost always it's something about the case that the group is anxious with, or disturbed by, or something parallel.

[Female, 20 years practice, 12 years in PSG]

I think that happens an awful lot, where someone is presenting a case, and they're doing exactly what the patient does. Like they'll talk about a patient rambling, and they'll be rambling too. It doesn't happen always, but it happens with fair regularity.

[Female, 40 years practice, 17 years in PSG]

Sometimes the group will start reacting in an uncharacteristic way, for example, very anxious, or making a lot of jokes, and it appears to be a reaction to the material being presented. Someone notices and remarks on it. Awareness of it can shed some light on the patient being discussed.

[Male, 30 years practice, 25 years in PSG]

I remember it being identified in the group when a presenter was talking about being really bored with his patient and the whole room shut down and started yawning.

[Male, 10 years practice, 3 years in PSG]

Sometimes it's a feeling of hopelessness. It happens more with patients who are *so* difficult. I have a colleague who presented her most difficult case, not just difficult but impossible, and nothing was ever going to happen with this man. And there the group was paralleling the hopeless/helpless feelings. This patient was out to make certain that nothing was ever going to happen in his life, and it never did. He finally stopped treatment.

[Female, 35 years practice, 15 years in PSG]

### My own experience

Sometimes when we are discussing a case, someone will point out that the group is reacting in an uncharacteristic way. We might be very anxious about a patient, when normally we're pretty calm. We might be having trouble paying attention, and small side conversations will keep breaking out. We try to use these observations as information about the patient, and it's often very useful because it can help explain the therapist's reactions in the treatment.

## Has the group ever told you that you shouldn't have done what you did?

Since members present their most difficult cases, it's almost inevitable that they will at times present their mistakes and most questionable behavior. Most groups seem to be able to find a way to address these errors without shaming the presenter. Most people said the group had never told them directly that they had made a mistake, but found gentler ways to imply it.

Our group tends not to relate that way. We're much more respectful of each other. We might say, "I wouldn't do that, I would have been tempted to do such-and-such." Maybe once or twice in the eleven years where something happened that's just very basic, like about confidentiality, someone did say that.

[Female, 25 years practice, 11 years in PSG]

We're all very PC about what we think people could have been doing differently, but we come from a "strength" perspective so we wouldn't have given feedback of that sort. I'm sure we all had felt it at some point, though.

[Female, 5 years practice, 1 year in PSG]

The monitor would catch someone who told you that. But you would know they thought that.

[Female, 30 years practice, 3 years in PSG]

Sometimes people will make a joke, or roll their eyes, like "Oh no! You didn't." I can be a little impetuous, or impulsive. I'll get a bright idea and I'll blurt it out, and they gently remind me to slow down.

[Female, 20 years practice, 12 years in PSG]

We're usually pretty sensitive, and we'll say, "It might have been better if you'd done this instead." You get the idea even though they haven't said it. It's not fun to hear it.

[Male, 10 years practice, 3 years in PSG]

When there's feedback given, there are certainly questions about what's making it difficult for the clinician to address an issue, or be more challenging. There are questions about one's approach only going so far, and what else might need to happen. It's said as "What else could you do? What aren't you doing?" There's challenge around thinking about all that stuff.

[Female, 25 years practice, 1 year in PSG]

We try not to be openly critical of each other. We might say, "How come you did that?"

[Female, 45 years practice, 30 years in PSG]

Others said that the group *had* told them that they shouldn't have done what they did, but that they felt safe enough to tolerate hearing it.

This group is so safe, and we all feel so understood, that it's okay, because I'm only presenting the most difficult people. If I was presenting a case that I thought was going fabulously and I felt really good about it, and they said "Why did you do *that*?" that would be very different. I would be questioning myself. But with these cases I know I'm not handling it well.

[Female, 35 years practice, 15 years in PSG]

I have a sense that has happened, when people said "Ouch! So how do we fix that?" I don't have a sense that it was punitive, but that it was collaborative, that we all make mistakes, so let's try to understand it and see how it can be managed.

[Male, 15 years practice, 1 year in PSG]

Sometimes people know before they even begin their case presentation that they've done something wrong.

I kind of knew it as I was telling it, or I wouldn't have brought it into the group. I wasn't surprised, and they don't say it in a shaming and punitive way, so it kind of confirms my own experience. It makes me feel I can trust them to be honest.

[Female, 25 years practice, 8 years in PSG]

I might say it myself, but I would say, "I would think about this another way," or "I would handle that differently." I don't think it's explicitly said, "Oh my God, you shouldn't have done that." There are other ways to make the point.

[Female, 35 years practice, 2 years in PSG]

They say, "I wouldn't do that. I would do this." It's much more likely that I'll say it myself. "Wait till you hear what I did!"

[Female, 35 years practice, 32 years in PSG]

If they've told me that, they never said it that way. They're almost too nice. They'll say, "Have you thought of doing it this way?" And because I am so direct, I'll say, "I think I made a mistake."

[Female, 20 years practice, 15 years in PSG]

We've all made mistakes, we've all done things that we wish we hadn't done, and it's for us to say that, not for someone else to judge what we've done. It's got to be safe.

[Female, 25 years practice, 15 years in PSG]

Sometimes when the group did give critical feedback it was difficult and painful to hear.

It feels pejorative when it's said that way. Many times it's not really the case, and later I wonder if I had presented it wrong.

[Female, 35 years practice, 30 years in PSG]

It's difficult to take that kind of criticism, but they're usually right so I don't do it again. I trust the group. Over all these years, they're like family.

[Female, 40 years practice, 18 years in PSG]

**My own experience**

Here's another question where I can say that it doesn't happen very often but it has happened. I can remember one situation where I was seeing a couple that had been referred by the woman's individual therapist, and I was in the process of getting into a big dispute with that other therapist about her treatment, when the group reined me in and helped me contain myself. I apologized to the other therapist, and we were better able to coordinate the two treatment situations.

# Discussion

I hope that, in any peer supervision group, anything a member wants to look at is fair game for the group. Even experienced clinicians can get stuck in countertransference reactions to patients. Even experienced clinicians can learn new approaches and techniques. Even the experienced therapist may get stuck—maybe not every week, but often enough, so that even the best therapist can use a peer supervision group to get the help he or she needs. No one is so experienced that they've seen everything before.

Freud called our work one of the "impossible professions"; there are so many places to slip up, to get stuck, to not know exactly what to do or say. Because we are human beings, we are imperfect. Being in a group with other clinicians can mitigate the shame of making errors, and can soften the blow to our narcissism. It may also help us navigate those situations where we have to make repairs with a patient.

The way in which cases are presented varies from group to group and from individual to individual, with no consensus about the proper way to do it. I think that almost any structure is acceptable as long as everyone agrees to it. There are advantages to planning, and advantages to spontaneity. Someone who knows in advance that he or she is presenting can organize the material more clearly than someone who presents on the fly. In every group, urgency takes precedence over prior arrangements, and this makes sense to me.

I think that sometimes presenters, in their anxiety, can get caught up in the facts, and overwhelm the group with information. At a professional convention a few years ago, I participated in a demonstration group where the presenter was not allowed to give any facts, only feelings, and the group was still able to provide powerful reactions and feedback, which for me made clear that the facts are not as important as we might sometimes think. It is also helpful when the person presenting a case

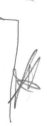

specifies what he or she wants from the group, as this will focus the discussion.

Frequency of presentation is almost irrelevant, as people get something out of the group even when they only listen and react. Some practices are more difficult than others; some therapists may even specialize in suicidal or otherwise challenging patients. These therapists might have more occasions to present difficult cases.

In some ways it's hard to imagine not being even a little nervous about bringing up a difficult case. The possibility of being shamed, even if the group is completely safe, always exists, depending on the degree of one's grandiosity or narcissism. One is already exposed as less than perfect by bringing in the case and asking for help. In a well-functioning group, this anxiety can be acknowledged and even discussed.

Everyone acknowledges that it's hard to hear that you made a mistake, especially when you know it's true. In a sense, that's exactly what we expect to hear when we present a case; otherwise it would be progressing normally and we wouldn't need to bring it into the group. It's rare that a group says directly "You really blew it there"; most groups are kinder and gentler than that. But we get the idea nonetheless. Hopefully we feel safe enough in the group to tolerate hearing it.

In the well-functioning and ideal group, there would be no need to censor or edit oneself. Anxiety about presenting would be part of the presentation. In the real world, we might not want to be exposed as doing something inept or questionable. It is a very positive sign that the vast majority of our interviewees are in groups where they feel safe enough not to have to conceal their work.

Obviously, especially in a large group, some suggestions are going to sound more appealing than others, but I think it's useful not to judge too quickly or to reject anything out of hand. This may be hard to do when it immediately feels off the mark. Staying open to all the feedback can be challenging, but I think it can open one up to new ideas and possibilities. Different people process information in different ways; there is no one right way.

In a large group, many different opinions can be confusing. If members share a theoretical orientation their comments will not range too far afield, and a consensus may be reached. But when there is no resolution it can be difficult to sit with the dissonance and tension of conflicting advice and suggestions.

Parallel process is an area where experience in groups and experience leading groups can be especially relevant. The phenomenon of parallel process can also occur in individual supervision, but it may be more easily visible in a group, where many different members may be reacting to the case presentation. It would be a loss if this information were overlooked or ignored, because it can shed so much light on the case, and may help unlock the puzzle of what is going wrong in the treatment.

# Chapter 7

# The Positive and the Negative

In this chapter we will look at some of the benefits of being in the group, as well as some of the drawbacks. We will address the rest of the group process issues: conflict, disagreement, and dislike, and how they feel about other members, some of which were addressed previously (feelings about absences and about social contact). The very survival of the group can depend how the group handles these issues.

We will also look at the ways a peer group differs from a regular supervision group. We will see what people like and dislike about the group experience, what people feel is missing, or if they are so unhappy that they are considering leaving the group.

## How would you describe what you get from the group?

There were a number of different aspects of the experience mentioned in response to this question. The most common response (sixteen people) was community, collegiality, and connection to other professionals. Fourteen people mentioned support, and another fourteen cited learning, continuing education, intellectual stimulation, and professional development. Ten people mentioned reassurance, validation, and normalizing of their experience. Nine people said they get help, and seven said they got insight. Five people each mentioned: holding and comfort; safety; and personal growth.

Many people find the group an antidote to the isolation of private practice.

> I feel very isolated in individual private practice. Even though there are a lot of therapists in my building, we're all very busy, and we tend to leave right away when we're done. We don't tend to sit in each other's

offices and talk about something that's bothering us about a case. For me, it's a lifeline.

[Female, 20 years practice, 15 years in PSG]

It's very isolating to do therapy, and most of my friends aren't therapists, so I'm not going to talk about what happened today in the office. It feels very good to be dealing with people who understand what you're dealing with all the time.

[Female, 40 years practice, 17 years in PSG]

It mitigates the feeling of professional isolation. Being around other professionals and sharing. I get other people's perspectives, which is useful, because it can be something I've missed completely.

[Female, 25 years practice, 20 years in PSG]

Private practice is very isolating. I'm in a solo office. I don't see anyone except patients all day, all week. It's important to have a group of colleagues I can just hang with, without having to think about and watch everything I say.

[Male, 30 years practice, 25 years in PSG]

For many people, peer group is an essential part of their professional lives. Many of the people interviewed have been in the same peer supervision group for many years, perhaps their entire professional career.

It's a sort of sustaining environment for me professionally and even personally, to know that every week I go someplace with a group of colleagues. Because of my connection with the hospital and the teaching environment there are other groups in my life, so I don't feel so isolated. But this is a more intensely connected group than the others.

[Female, 35 years practice, 15 years in PSG]

I don't know where I'd be without it.

[Female, 20 years practice, 15 years in PSG]

People usually feel supported by the group in their work with clients. The group forms a safety net that contains the anxiety generated by a difficult patient.

One of the main things is it helps bind my own anxiety in life, of having a practice and worrying about patients who are in trouble, and worrying about whether I'm doing a good job with them or not. I tend to be an anxious person in general, and it's tremendously comforting to know that, whatever goes on, there's a place to talk about it that's comfortable and helpful. I feel enormous trust in the group. They're really good clinicians, so I know that, whatever's going on, I'll get some help.

When I have specific questions I always end up with more ideas or more insight.

[Female, 25 years practice, 11 years in PSG]

It's also important to have a backup system, so I know that if I encounter something difficult or distressing I can go and talk about and get the help I need.

[Male, 30 years practice, 25 years in PSG]

I get the holding, and knowing there's a place to discuss any of the cases I'm working with. If anyone's percolating very harshly, then I know I can't wait to go and talk about that case. It's like a therapy session: even if you don't have anything specific to say, you know that you have that anchor.

[Male, 15 years practice, 5 years in PSG]

Whenever I bring up a patient I'm feeling some difficulty with it's always been helpful, because it gets rid of a lot of that tension, just to talk about it. It's not even that someone is suggesting something so terrific. It's more just talking about it in a safe environment, and having people hear the difficulty. It's more the process of presenting than the feedback. There are suggestions that people make that are helpful, because it opens up something, but it's more the safety of being able to talk about it and feel that it's normalized. It's a way of discharging some energy that would get in the way.

[Female, 40 years practice, 17 years in PSG]

I get some professional reassurance, validation, affirmation that I do know what I'm doing, even though I sometimes feel like I don't. Everybody struggles, because it's hard, and sometimes painful. Especially when you feel hopeless, and sometimes it is hopeless, and that's hard to accept, that you can't have an impact.

[Female, 20 years practice, 7 years in PSG]

Some people found the group normalized their own experience.

Hearing that others had emotional reactions to their patients was very reassuring.

[Female, 40 years practice, 15 years in PSG]

It's nice to be in a collegial professional setting, with people who are doing the same work that I'm doing, and are also facing the same struggles and difficulties at times that I'm having. I feel that I'm not alone, that what I'm experiencing is not different than what other therapists are experiencing.

[Male, 40 years practice, 8 months in PSG]

Many people mentioned the feeling of safety.

> It's a sense of safety, of being with peers who acknowledge the difficulty of what we're all doing, and there's some security in talking about something that's tricky, and hearing what everyone else would do. Very often, people will talk about something I haven't thought of, but we're all pretty much on the same wavelength with patients. There's a kind of security in hearing that I'm basically on the right track. There's a lot of reassurance.
>
> [Female, 40 years practice, 17 years in PSG]

> I get a sense of security that if something really bothers me I have a place to go and take it, and if I feel that I'm at sea, I know that in one or two weeks I will be able to talk about this, and I'll have the security of people whose opinion I trust. I trust the group members. I think they're good therapists, good clinicians, and they're ideas are valuable, very valuable.
>
> [Female, 20 years practice, 12 years in PSG]

People in a peer supervision group get challenged intellectually, and the group can be a place for continuing education and ongoing learning.

> I get a kind of supervision that feels really safe. I get new ideas. I find myself saying often, "I wouldn't have thought to do that, or say it that way. I wouldn't have thought of going that route. This is very helpful." Another person in the group has a way of reaching an outcome a lot quicker than I would, and I like that, too.
>
> [Female, 20 years practice, 15 years in PSG]

> The people in the group are smart, and tuned in, and we're appreciative of each other's angles, that they're really helpful. It both reinforces what I do and also it's a place to ask the questions that most bother me about how I'm working and having others resonate with my dilemma. I'm not alone, it's not my inadequacies.
>
> [Female, 25 years practice, 1 year in PSG]

> I believe that it enriches me because it keeps me learning. And I believe that the most important thing in my life at this point [of being 80] is not to close myself off to the surrounding realities of my life, one of the most important of which is teaching and learning.
>
> [Male, 40 years practice, 7 years in PSG]

> It's very helpful intellectually, to get me to think about new things, things I can't get to on my own.
>
> [Female, 25 years practice, 15 years in PSG]

I learn, which is wonderful, and even if it's not necessarily new information maybe it's a new way of looking at something, a new perspective that I didn't think of. Even though I'm not presenting a case I can still learn from the person who's presenting and from the comments of the other members. I also like that I can contribute something, and maybe help that person, or support them, reaffirm his or her perspective on the case.

[Male, 40 years practice, 8 months in PSG]

For some people, peer group is a place for personal growth.

There have been health crises in my family, and the group was terrific. Other people in the group also have health issues and we talk about all that. There's a lot of emotional support. And then it gets woven into what we're doing as clinicians. Our growth and development as therapists is part of our growth and development as people, so that's beautifully woven into the fabric of the group.

[Male, 38 years practice, 15 years in PSG]

It's a safe place to explore some personal questions as a therapist, where I'm not going to be judged. It's also useful to hear all the other perspectives, where I was on track, where I was off track, how I might have gotten back on track.

[Female, 25 years practice, 8 years in PSG]

For many, the social and professional network the group creates is extremely valuable.

I get support, not just in my work, but in my life, my various life crises. The group has been there for me.

[Female, 45 years practice, 30 years in PSG]

I get a sense of collegial connection. I feel like I really belong to the group. I feel that we have something really special in the way that we're working together. I like everyone in the group and feel very connected to them. It is a priority for me. It's important because the work is so difficult, and I do feel the need for contact and support.

[Female, 30 years practice, 8 months in PSG]

It's a feeling of community, and support, and of having colleagues available, even outside of group time, colleagues I could call and I would trust their judgment and their knowledge of me and my way of practice.

[Female, 30 years practice, 30 years in PSG]

For some the variety of opinions and different points of view is very important.

I've always preferred it to the idea of having an individual supervisor, because I want different points of view.

[Female, 20 years practice, 15 years in PSG]

I find it so nourishing to hear other people's perspectives and experiences. It's also a bit intimidating, because I always wonder if I'm not good enough.

[Female, 5 years practice, 1 year in PSG]

One person remarked on the comfort he got from the way the group approached the problems of the work.

It reassures me that there are good people out there trying to do this work with integrity, and trying to manage things like burnout and frustration honestly, and not just pretending they don't exist.

[Male, 15 years practice, 1 year in PSG]

### My own experience

Let me say again that one of the pleasures of doing this book was hearing how much most of the people interviewed get from their peer groups. I myself am one of those people. We participate in each other's lives in so many ways, beyond merely professional relationships. We attend parties, weddings, and funerals together. We also turn to each other for support in our personal and professional lives. I can't imagine not having them in my life.

# What's missing from your group experience?

As much as most of the interviewees enjoyed their groups, there was often something missing in their experience. Only four people said there was nothing missing. Lack of focus and the wish for more structure was mentioned most often (seven people). Six people said they wanted the group to do more processing of its own dynamics. Five people said they wanted the group to be larger, or to have more members of the opposite sex. Four people said they wished the group to meet more often, or for a longer time. Another four people said they wanted more expertise and/or authority. One person mentioned wishing to feel more connected to the other group members, and another wished to feel safer. Let's start with the people who wanted more structure.

I would like it to be more structured. And sometimes people talk over each other and that becomes confusing.

[Female, 25 years practice, 8 years in PSG]

I guess sometimes when the group gets very distracted into the personal chitchat. I mind that. I would prefer we didn't do that. I'd prefer we fulfill the purpose. But I don't always want to take a role in making that happen.

[Female, 25 years practice, 15 years in PSG]

Sometimes it can feel unfocused. I hate talking about politics, and we do a lot of that.

[Male, 30 years practice, 25 years in PSG]

We've talked occasionally about following a train of thought. Maybe one week something will open up that we all find fascinating, like a theoretical issue, and we don't necessarily follow up on it. Sometimes a paper or a book will interest us, but we don't have the time for that usually.

[Female, 25 years practice, 15 years in PSG]

Meeting monthly was a problem for some people.

I wish we met more often. We can call each other between meetings, but it's happened rarely. If something is really urgent. If I had a colleague next door, I'd just go to their office, and I'd prefer that to the phone.

[Female, 20 years practice, 15 years in PSG]

Some people wanted to be more engaged in the group.

It's not enough time. I'd like to meet more often for a little longer, and do more work on how the work impacts us emotionally.

[Female, 30 years practice, 8 months in PSG]

It's my own problem, in that I don't get together with them enough socially. I live in a different part of town and I don't call people enough, or go to lunch.

[Female, 40 years practice, 18 years in PSG]

I guess what's missing is more continuity, more time, more keeping track of one another's group experiences over time, following up and seeing how things evolve, and knowing each other's cases and groups and hold them in a richer way, but I'm not willing at this point to commit to the time that would take.

[Male, 15 years practice, 1 year in PSG]

Some groups need more diversity.

> I sometimes worry that we all know each other so well now that we're missing something. Also we all come from a similar theoretical orientation, and four out of five were trained at the same institute. I sometimes worry that we're missing someone with a very different point of view.
> [Female, 25 years practice, 11 years in PSG]

This person wanted *less* diversity.

> I wish there were a more consistent group of people. It's a wide spectrum of therapeutic orientations represented, and it makes for more confusion than for stimulating points of view.
> [Male, 10 years practice, 3 years in PSG]

Some groups felt too small.

> I wish that a few more people would join.
> [Female, 35 years practice, 30 years in PSG]

Someone from a group that was all women had this to say.

> None of us would feel the need to have a man join us just to balance the group. We're all happily married, we have men in our lives, but there is something missing. It would change the dynamic.
> [Female, 20 years practice, 7 years in PSG]

Some people wanted more expertise.

> I want the hierarchy of having an expert to give us their lens of experience.
> [Female, 5 years practice, 1 year in PSG]

> We were all neophytes, and we all thought we could have benefited from an expert. At times it was the blind leading the blind.
> [Female, 30 years practice, 3 years in PSG]

> There are only a couple of people there who have taught me anything.
> [Female, 25 years practice, 20 years in PSG]

Many groups don't do enough processing of what goes on in the group.

> Perhaps what's missing is a little bit more of group dynamics, talking about what's happening between me and another person, or what's happening in the group itself.
> [Female, 30 years practice, 30 years in PSG]

There are areas that are unstated among us, which would make us move more into a T-group or group therapy kind of thing. The missing pieces of being able to say directly to someone, "I think the way you talk about that, you have a problem with it." "I feel unsupported when this or that happens." We do a little of that, but not a lot.

[Male, 40 years practice, 15 years in PSG]

There's a part of me that feels it should get more personal, in terms of the group interaction, not outside issues but the process of the group. We don't talk about process very often, and I don't think we're very good at it. We do it only when we have to, and when we've done it, it's only gotten us into trouble.

[Female, 40 years practice, 17 years in PSG]

We don't do the emotional processing that we do in my therapy group.

[Female, 35 years practice, 5 years in PSG]

For some people the group was not knowledgeable about certain areas, such as couple counseling, or running therapy groups.

Because I'm craving to learn how to go to a deeper level than I do, it would be interesting to have someone with a psychoanalytic orientation for that kind of rich perspective.

[Female, 10 years practice, 6 years in PSG]

At the time no one knew how to treat couples, so we would occasionally try to talk about it but that was the weakest area.

[Female, 40 years practice, 15 years in PSG]

No one else was able to give knowledgeable feedback about groups.

[Male, 15 years practice, 5 years in PSG]

For this person, a feeling of safety was missing.

I wish there was more questioning rather than judgment making. Sometimes someone says something and people get on a bandwagon and it starts to feel like a total attack. I wish it felt safer.

[Female, 35 years practice, 30 years in PSG]

## My own experience

A short while ago I would have said that what was missing from my own group was process: the conscious and deliberate discussion and examination of the group itself. But recently the group agreed to set aside the last fifteen minutes of group time to do that. I'm excited that we're including this aspect of group dynamics, and hope that it will make the group even more rewarding.

## How is a peer group different from a group with a leader?

People seek out a peer group, rather than a group led by someone specific, usually an experienced and expert clinician. What differences do people see that go into that choice?

Many people liked being responsible for the way the group functions, rather than giving that responsibility over to the leader.

> The responsibility falls on us. It's a question of owning one's place in the room. In a led group the leadership is given to the leader, whether they're paid or not. It allows for an outside observing ego to emerge, to discuss the dynamics and process of the group.
>
> [Male, 15 years practice, 5 years in PSG]

> We each have to take ownership of the process, and the frame. We also need to take ownership of asking for what we need. It's a different quality of responsibility. I feel a need to watch more carefully. In a curious way, you can't be so self-involved, because you have to be holding the whole group in mind.
>
> [Female, 35 years practice, 2 years in PSG]

> It puts more responsibility on the group members, to grow up in a certain way. The group supervisors I've seen have had agendas of their own and purposes for the group that structure it in a way that may not work for me. When you have a peer group, the group has to evolve itself, and take responsibility for that, which is a learning process.
>
> [Female, 20 years practice, 12 years in PSG]

Several people acknowledged that the peer group had to work harder at staying focused on the task, and on maintaining the functioning in general.

> I think we're always struggling with trying to define who we are, what the purpose is, are we going to use time to talk about marketing and, if we are, how are we going to do it. There's a conflict between the clinical aspect and the business aspect of the group.
>
> [Female, 30 years practice, 8 months in PSG]

Some people didn't want to pay for supervision, or to remain in the role of student. For some people, it feels analogous to the difference between being a child and being an adult.

> The notion of "peer" and the absence of turning to a higher authority confirm a certain maturation. And the quality of being safe without a leader is pretty remarkable. That has enriched the experience, that we all share responsibility for that, instead of giving it over to the authority.
>
> [Male, 40 years practice, 15 years in PSG]

> At a certain point in your career, you have to step up and take responsibility for what you do. You can't be a child forever. In acting they call it "taking your space." You stake your claim to what you do. Peer supervision is part of that.
>
> [Male, 30 years practice, 25 years in PSG]

> After twenty or thirty years of doing the work, the problems I encounter aren't due to not knowing how to do something, so they don't require an expert to teach me something. They have to do with needing another point of view from outside the system of the patient and me. I can get that from my peers. Going to a paid supervisor feels infantilizing.
>
> [Male, 30 years practice, 25 years in PSG]

> We're all therapists with a number of years of experience under our belt, so we've been in the field for a long time, and at this stage we don't need to have a leader directing the group. We're experienced enough, seasoned enough, to participate in a group ourselves. It's an affirmation of who we are as therapists.
>
> [Male, 40 years practice, 8 months in PSG]

> Peer group feels more respectful to me as a senior therapist. This is not to say that I couldn't learn at a conference from somebody who was giving a lecture. I can do that, but I wouldn't want that every other week.
>
> [Female, 25 years practice, 15 years in PSG]

> At one point when I was younger I would have enjoyed a led group, if I could find a leader that I liked, but I don't feel that way so much anymore. I feel at my age that I don't need a led group. I would be the person leading the group.
>
> [Female, 40 years practice, 17 years in PSG]

Some people found the presence of a leader inhibiting, or otherwise problematic.

There's more freedom and less worry about what the supervisor's going to think.

[Female, 30 years practice, 30 years in PSG]

I can be more honest, because I have a thing with authority, that I want the leader to be thinking well of me. So I'd be cautious about how I presented myself.

[Female, 35 years practice, 32 years in PSG]

I love groups and I love being a leader of my groups, but I hate being a member of a led group. My unresolved issues with authority, and with visibility and invisibility, and with shame and exposure, all those get really triggered in a group with a leader. If I'm not comfortable with the leader I tend to go silent, and it's really not productive for me.

[Male, 10 years practice, 6 months in PSG]

I feel less inhibited in a peer group because there's no authority figure.

[Female, 24 years practice, 20 years in PSG]

Peer group is less competitive. When there's a leader people compete for attention.

[Female, 40 years practice, 18 years in PSG]

For some it's a question of the power that resides in the leader.

There's no agenda in a peer group. I've been in groups where I was going to learn somebody's way of working, but I also felt it was too dogmatic, too authoritarian. It depends on how much they have an agenda to promote their way of thinking and ideology.

[Female, 25 years practice, 1 year in PSG]

I didn't have a secure feeling with the leader. It was more clinical and academic. So there was more concern with how I was going to present a case. I had more concern about the leader's judgments, and I didn't like that.

[Female, 35 years practice, 30 years in PSG]

Peer group is much more egalitarian. There's no power differential, and it's much easier to accept feedback. There's less anxiety because you don't feel you're being scolded or shamed.

[Male, 45 years practice, 20 years in PSG]

There's a more democratic focus in a peer group. If the leader is there, you present to the leader. There's no way around that. The leader sets the tone.

[Female, 40 years practice, 15 years in PSG]

I didn't like the supervisor thing. It felt authoritarian.

[Female, 20 years practice, 15 years in PSG]

Others said they preferred the freedom of a peer group.

Peer group is everyone on the same level, while the group with a leader isn't. The leader has a plan and determines the direction and structure of the group. He has an agenda.

[Male, 40 years practice, 7 years in PSG]

In peer group there's no agenda. You make of it what you wish, instead of someone telling you what it should be. It really feels more adult than having a leader.

[Female, 45 years practice, 30 years in PSG]

People like the equality they experience in a peer group.

We all felt we had something of value to share, so there wasn't one person who was "the expert."

[Female, 30 years practice, 3 years in PSG]

You're being taught in a led group, and it has advantages and disadvantages. You're learning from someone who supposedly has more skill and knowledge in a particular area, but I think it does inhibit group members from feeling that they have as much to offer.

[Female, 40 years practice, 17 years in PSG]

A few people thought a led group functioned better.

I think it gets rid of a lot of the neurotic group interaction. The group leader can call it much quicker than in a peer group, where sometimes it's not called at all. Also, I think you can get into the theory better.

[Female, 35 years practice, 30 years in PSG]

The led group is more structured, and there is less crosstalk.

[Female, 25 years practice, 8 years in PSG]

Without a leader there's no one to keep the group on track.

[Male, 45 years practice, 5 years in PSG]

Surprisingly, group leaders are not always good at leading.

I'm also in a group with a leader. In the peer group we can actually deal with the dynamics that come up with and for us, rather than having to push them aside and pretend that they're not there. I find that anytime I'm in a group and the group process is not attended to, and one is not authorized to attend to it, it's really damaging. In the led group, there's lip service being paid to attending to it, but it's really not paid attention to and it's been really problematic, to the extent that I'm not sure how long I want to continue in the led group.

[Male, 15 years practice, 1 year in PSG]

In one group, I didn't like the leader's style, in that he perceived himself as democratic, but that was not my experience of him. He felt quite free to tell me about myself in ways that I found wounding at times, so I left.

[Female, 25 years practice, 15 years in PSG]

Some of the leaders I've had over the years have been very good with group process, and some are much less skilled with groups. I was in one where the leader had no idea how to handle the group process at all. He never brought it up. People would take digs at each other and it was never addressed.

[Female, 25 years practice, 10 years in PSG]

I was in a supervision group with a leader recently, where I paid her, and I did not like it and I dropped out. I didn't feel it was worth it. She had a lot of expertise in her area, but she wasn't that good. I don't like having to defer to someone who I may or may not think is on my wavelength, or knows as much as I do, or is as intuitive as I am, or works the way I do. I joined that group because of her expertise, but it very soon degenerated into a kind of peer group, and she kept having to have the last word.

[Female, 20 years practice, 7 years in PSG]

Even in a peer group a leader can sometimes emerge.

At one point, there was someone who was sort of the elder statesman, but that really wasn't helpful, because there was a sense of hierarchical structure.

[Male, 45 years practice, 20 years in PSG]

## My own experience

For me, the peer group is completely different from a led group. I love that there is no power differential, and that we are ourselves responsible for the functioning of the group. I know I am an experienced clinician, among other experienced clinicians, none of whom needs to be told what to do. I feel like an adult in a group of adults, rather than a child with a parent. I ask for help when I need it, and give help when asked and when I have something useful to say.

# Has there ever been overt conflict? How are conflicts resolved?

At some point, most groups experience conflict among two or more of the members. How these conflicts are managed and processed can determine whether the group survives. A willingness to address and contain conflict is crucial.

Overall, twenty-six people said there had been conflict in the group. Only eight people said there had never been overt conflict in their group, and four of those were people who had been in their group less than a year, so perhaps had not been there long enough to have observed or participated in a conflictual situation.

Some groups seem to have difficulty dealing with open conflict.

Two of the newer members have this big conflict. What it's about I have no idea. It's deep in their psyches, and it's not really about the group. I think it's about something within these two people. They trigger each other in a very bad way. The group tried to handle it, but we're not a therapy group so I don't think we could get deep enough into it. I don't think it's an appropriate place to get into what's really going on with them.

[Female, 25 years practice, 15 years in PSG]

Another member was confronted about her inability to make a commitment to the group and she got extremely defensive. It was useless. Whenever conflict has arisen, nothing has come out of it.

[Female, 25 years practice, 20 years in PSG]

It was a pretty passive group. There were several people in the group who avoided conflict in general.

[Female, 5 years practice, 1 year in PSG]

I've had one situation, where there was a lot of conflict with another woman. My situation is about 85 percent resolved. Mostly conflicts get pushed under the rug.

[Female, 40 years practice, 18 years in PSG]

One time I got into a strong disagreement with another member about a clinical issue, and another member tried to smooth it over so we wouldn't disagree. That didn't feel useful.

[Male, 30 years practice, 25 years in PSG]

I've gotten very angry with another member about a certain judgmental quality that I was just fed up with. I don't think it was processed enough. It's more a case of time healing all wounds.

[Female, 35 years practice, 30 years in PSG]

Sometimes the conflict is about how the group itself is functioning.

I have often felt that the group gets so involved with each other and their spouses that you have to say very loudly, "I have something to present," or it gets glossed over and time goes by, and we're talking about vacations, and movies, which for me is a waste of time.

[Female, 35 years practice, 30 years in PSG]

I brought up an issue that I wasn't getting what I wanted out of the group, that they don't stay on task, they start late, that people are not committed to being here, and I don't want this to be the quality of the group. And they got very quiet, and nobody said anything.

[Female, 25 years practice, 20 years in PSG]

Sometimes the conflict occurs when one group member uses personal information as a weapon against another. This group tried to anticipate some issues, but it may have backfired.

In one group we presented our own genograms, so people would know our family-of-origin issues, but you can't use that information as ammunition. When people got hurt they would sometimes resort to using that information in a negative way.

[Female, 35 years practice, 2 years in PSG]

There was an instance where another member and I did have a fight, and I threatened to leave. She had asked me to see a family member of a patient of hers, and I didn't want to because I thought the situation needed a family therapist, and I didn't feel qualified. I was also concerned about the father and the potential for violence. And she was kind of dismissive of my concerns. And she said, "What's the matter? Was your mother abusive?" The fact is my mother was abusive, and she knew that because we were close friends and I had told her. This was right in front of a new group member, and I said, "No. I just think there's trouble brewing." But I was furious. She was revealing my personal stuff in front of this stranger. She called me the next day to apologize, but I said it made me feel not safe to be there, and that I was thinking about leaving the group. She said, "I can't believe you would do that."

[Female, 35 years practice, 32 years in PSG]

To this person, addressing the issue did not appear to help, and seemed to actually make things worse.

> I'm thinking of the fight between two of the women, where I thought they were both inappropriate. It played itself out, it was eventually okay, but I think that when we talked about it, it made it escalate more.
>
> [Female, 40 years practice, 17 years in PSG]

Newly formed groups may consciously and intentionally avoid dealing with conflict.

> We're not dealing with that right now. We have so little time that we're focusing only on the clinical material. There was an issue between two people about an issue outside the group, and they settled it outside the group.
>
> [Female, 30 years practice, 8 months in PSG]

Some groups seem to be better at arriving at a resolution.

> At one time two of the women who are very close had a bit of a rift, and we were concerned that would affect the group. One of the people had told me that she felt more distant. There was some misunderstanding. We tried to help them talk it out in the group, and they also had a few phone conversations outside the group, and it ended up working out quite well.
>
> [Female, 25 years practice, 11 years in PSG]

> We say, "I'm feeling triggered," or "That was kind of icky," or "Yuck!" We'll look at each other and go, "What was *that*?" Sometimes someone's been really injured, or feels misunderstood, and that's no laughing matter. We've never not gotten to a good place.
>
> [Female, 25 years practice, 15 years in PSG]

> There have been a couple of situations where one person felt insulted or slighted by another. Someone always steps into the role of moderating the discussion and mediating the aggression.
>
> [Male, 30 years practice, 25 years in PSG]

> We're a very good group at talking about tensions as they arise. We don't do it a lot, but any time that we have to, we will.
>
> [Female, 25 years practice, 11 years in PSG]

> Somebody felt they weren't being heard or understood, or someone was judging them or making generalizations about them. We mirror the two people involved, and they go into a dialogue with each other. There's

an understanding that takes place. The issues don't go away because those are the issues of those people, but the energy is resolved.

[Female, 25 years practice, 8 years in PSG]

What's interesting to me is that usually the conflict does not involve the entire group. It's almost always an electricity between two individuals. What makes for an effective group is the capacity of those two people to look at their own stuff. When there's been conflict, the way we've been able to work with it is to have the individuals look at what this is stirring up for them. Often it's projection, or it's disappointment of expectations, or competition, a kind of rivalry, for time, for space, for recognition.

[Female, 35 years practice, 2 years in PSG]

Sometimes there's a little countertransference between the people in the group. Somehow we always manage to work it out. People somehow get beyond it. They apologize, or work it out. It depends on the situation. It doesn't continue growing into something that would fracture the group.

[Female, 45 years practice, 30 years in PSG]

One person and I are really dear friends, but I think I have angered her over the years. She hasn't angered me but I think I've pissed her off a couple of times. Naturally we all step in to make sure that everything is all right. If I said something in a harsh way, I try to explain it. Someone might say to me that I need to be more sensitive, because I can be a little harsh, and it gets resolved.

[Female, 35 years practice, 30 years in PSG]

There were a couple of times when people felt they were being criticized. More came out afterwards, they said something to another person in the group and it came back to them. And then the group addressed it, but in a more general way without naming the individual. One person brought it up and said, "I think there's a tendency to be critical sometimes. It's easy to be that way, is there a way we can guard against it for future sessions so people can feel safe?"

[Male, 10 years practice, 3 years in PSG]

In some cases the conflict was not resolved and one or more people left the group, although the remainder of the group continued to meet.

Two people met for coffee before the group and came in a half-hour late, not being aware of the time. That was the beginning of the feeling that one of them was enacting something. The one who left made it hard to talk about it, because of what she said, which was kind of arrogant, and there was no opportunity to talk about it. She left via a phone message.

[Female, 25 years practice, 1 year in PSG]

I was new to the group, and two of the women had a history of conflictual relationship. So I'm sitting there and they're blasting each other. But only one other person in the group leads groups, and it seemed that they had no idea how to handle it. I didn't know them well enough to understand what it was about. Both the women left, they both dropped out. I was surprised. It was not pleasant.

[Male, 15 years practice, 5 years in PSG]

The woman who invited me into the group did not have the same orientation as the rest of us, and that led to some conflict. When the rest of us were focusing on some of the emotional communications that would be effective, she wouldn't like them at all. She would come at it very cognitively and be very aggressive toward what we were doing. It wasn't working that well. We were all reacting to how controlling she was and we decided that it would be better to rotate the meetings. She decided to drop out.

[Female, 35 years practice, 5 years in PSG]

Two women got into arguments a lot. The first person who left, we all shared concerns about her capacity to do first-rate work. There was a kind of shallowness and rigidity that intersected with her obvious unattended-to health crisis. So she felt judged, and complained about feeling unsupported, and she announced one day that she wasn't coming anymore. We didn't process it with her. In the other case, there were muted fights. I guess the resolution in both cases was their departure.

[Male, 40 years practice, 15 years in PSG]

Directly addressing conflict can be frightening, even for experienced therapists.

It's almost as if we don't think the group could feed us for long if we had a lot of that going on. Maybe it's true. That part of it feels a little dangerous.

[Female, 40 years practice, 17 years in PSG]

I have some fear, probably going back to my childhood, that, left alone, siblings will kill each other, that total mayhem will break out without a leader, but that's never happened.

[Female, 25 years practice, 11 years in PSG]

I don't know that conflicts are resolved in the group, more that they're resolved with time. I can't say that I've experienced the group working those conflicts through so that I felt we had found a way of dealing with it. It's more like there's conflict, and there's so much pull not to do anything to upset the balance of the group that we go into a kind of denial about it. But we put it in a drawer for a while, on the back burner, and maybe never get to it again.

[Female, 40 years practice, 17 years in PSG]

There's a degree of resistance to discussing the process and dynamics in the group, or even a lack of awareness of those dynamics.

[Male, 15 years practice, 5 years in PSG]

In other cases the group did not survive the failure to resolve the conflict.

Too often the conflicts were not resolved, and ultimately it was a contributing factor to the demise of the group.

[Female, 35 years practice, 2 years in PSG]

Some people mentioned some interesting specific situations.

I actually got into a tiff with another group member, which got resolved adequately, I think. We socialized out of the group, and maybe that wasn't good for us. I think there was a misunderstanding about the depth of our friendship. She felt I was rejecting. The group tried to stay steady and inclusive of both of us. At one point the other person said she might drop out, and said she was uncomfortable in the group, and the group encouraged her to stick it out. Someone said, "It's not a good idea to kill off a member," which was a good way to phrase it. The person did stick it out and it was good for the group to go through a conflict where they didn't lose a member.

[Female, 20 years practice, 12 years in PSG]

The other man used to provoke one of the women intentionally, because he had issues from his family, and she was a soft object. I didn't interfere, but one of the other women stepped in and asked why he was picking on her. I don't think it's fully resolved.

[Male, 45 years practice, 5 years in PSG]

One time someone was talking about a patient, he had some complaints about things that were happening with the patient, and another member started to give advice, and said that these things happen, and he got furious. He said, "I want to have a place where I can express my anger, not to analyze it or be talked out of it."

[Male, 40 years practice, 7 years in PSG]

Someone was talking about a reaction she was having to a patient, and another member said, "It sounds like you need to be in your own private supervision, or even back in therapy." She got all bent out of shape, and very defensive. I think the healthier response might have been, "Maybe you have a point there. Why am I having this reaction to the patient?" I didn't think it was said as an attack, but it got interpreted that way.

[Female, 25 years practice, 20 years in PSG]

**My own experience**

I have seen groups disintegrate because resentments and conflicts were not processed. I once left a group where I was too often in conflict with another member, and where the group ethos was too different from my own. I never felt fully part of that group, and never felt safe enough to fully reveal myself or my work.

In the current group, I have rarely felt in conflict with anyone. I have gotten into disagreements with a few people about clinical issues, and some got a little heated. Other members sometimes get into conflicts with each other. These situations seem to be resolved, although they may just be dormant—it can be hard to tell.

# Is there anyone in the group you often disagree with?

The interviewees were fairly evenly divided on this question, sixteen saying that there was no one in the group they often disagreed with and eighteen saying that there was. But almost everyone mentioned some issue that regularly came up with another member.

For some, disagreements arose out of a personality issue.

One of the men can be obsessive with details, and if he presents a case it's influenced by the old medical model of presentation, and that's both training and characterological, and he can get lost in all those details. So part of the work of the group is managing that, on the one hand, and also we try to work with him to help him not do that, not just because it isn't a good use of our group, but because it isn't a good use of him. It's not how he can best work with his group, to be focused on all that minutia.

[Male, 15 years practice, 1 year in PSG]

One person gets off the subject sometimes, into an individualized trance, and people have to bring her back to the issue at hand.

[Female, 45 years practice, 30 years in PSG]

There's a woman in the group, and I really love her, and I understand how hard her life has been. I get the urgency. But sometimes it drives me crazy. Someone's talking and she'll suddenly interrupt, and it twists my head around. I don't want to hear about that now. It's not relevant. We really have a hard time saying it to each other, when that happens. Maybe it's hard because we all know each other so long that we accept the craziness, and we don't try to change something that's probably not changeable. Maybe that's also part of the acceptance of the group, but for me it requires a shutting down.

[Female, 40 years practice, 17 years in PSG]

There was someone years back who left that was a little righteous about what she knew.

[Female, 35 years practice, 30 years in PSG]

There was a period where we were very concerned with the member who was having a chronic illness and was dealing with it by being full of denial, super-positive, suppressing all the aggression. We were very concerned about how to help bring some of that to the fore but respect the defenses.

[Female, 35 years practice, 5 years in PSG]

This one person is a little sharp sometimes. The rest of us go with the flow and don't really confront her. Nobody addresses it directly. It's not a real conflict. If I really disagreed I would speak up. But it wouldn't be a conflict, it would just be a disagreement. We don't confront her because she's got her own problems, and she's kind of vulnerable. She's terrific in every other respect, so we tolerate it and protect her.

[Female, 20 years practice, 7 years in PSG]

There was another woman who didn't seem to be very well analyzed and didn't have her own individual therapy and was always coming in very needy and trying to monopolize the group. I was very glad when she left.

[Female, 35 years practice, 5 years in PSG]

Sometimes the problem was differing styles.

There are two people with whose presentations I find myself struggling. One is sometimes so direct and filled with critical affect that I get uncomfortable. The other gets too flowery and too intellectual, and his comments are too filled with theoretical stuff. Sometimes I say, "Get to the point."

[Male, 40 years practice, 15 years in PSG]

There are some competitive feelings in the group that I feel sometimes. In debate of things, who's right and who's wrong. We all have a more or less similar clinical approach, but there are definite differences in style, or how slow, how patiently, we might go.

[Female, 25 years practice, 1 year in PSG]

There are people in the group whose clinical opinions I don't respect. Someone is a concrete thinker who I don't respect. There are also a couple of people who use modalities I'm not comfortable with, which is different from saying they're not skilled clinicians.

[Male, 15 years practice, 5 years in PSG]

There is one woman who tends to be a little too dogmatic. I've said that to her.

[Male, 40 years practice, 7 years in PSG]

There's one person who has more of the "social worker" take on things. I'm not a social worker and I don't think that way, and I'm not interested in that, and I reject some of what she says, and I wish she were more psychoanalytic.

[Female, 25 years practice, 15 years in PSG]

It's more a matter of style than content. She tends to see things as if they are right or wrong, rather than from a certain vantage point. I find that kind of alienating.

[Female, 10 years practice, 6 years in PSG]

For some people, the issue was clinical competence.

There's one woman I'm very cautious about. I'm not sure about her training. When she talks about patients it doesn't sound like she has had any real training. I don't think she's appropriate for the group.

[Male, 45 years practice, 5 years in PSG]

It's very frustrating These are people who've been in the field for twenty-five or thirty years, and I wonder what they've been doing for all that time.

[Female, 25 years practice, 20 years in PSG]

There are some people whose clinical judgment I question.

[Male, 30 years practice, 25 years in PSG]

For the most part, I trust everyone in the group, and I would refer a patient to almost everyone, but there are people in the group I would not refer anyone to. That feels bad. I don't want to feel that way about them, and I feel guilty.

[Female, 40 years practice, 17 years in PSG]

A few people were able to recognize that the problem was more their own, and tried to contain the feelings.

> I'm very quick to judgment; I like to make snap judgments, so I say to myself, "Here I go again. Chill out! Maybe there's something to what they're saying."
>
> [Female, 30 years practice, 30 years in PSG]

> There was a person, but over the course of time, because I was follow-ing the agreements of the group, part of which was to be nonjudgmental and open, I found that the person did have something to offer, too. And that really did work.
>
> [Female, 30 years practice, 3 years in PSG]

## My own experience

I have encountered this situation, of being in group with someone I kept disagreeing with, a couple of times. In one case, it was so intense that it led to my almost leaving the group. Fortunately, the other person left first. In the other case, we accepted the differences and moved on. I don't have to agree with everyone all the time.

# Is there anyone in the group you don't like?

Only five people said that there was now or had been someone in their group that they just didn't like. For some people it isn't a big problem.

> My nature is to shift the focus rather than confront it.
>
> [Female, 25 years practice, 15 years in PSG]

> It has been true in the past. It was a little uncomfortable, but because the group is so large it really didn't matter.
>
> [Female, 35 years practice, 30 years in PSG]

> Over the course of the group I became more accepting.
>
> [Female, 30 years practice, 3 years in PSG]

But for others the situation can be hard to tolerate or to resolve.

> There was someone who the group had a problem with. It was a perso-nality issue that made it hard to keep her in the group. This person had an intensity, and because she was so intense she kept interrupting. She couldn't hear what was going on, and she couldn't contain herself, which was very frustrating to the people who were presenting, and to the rest of us, because we couldn't get a word in edgewise. It wasn't the

trusting, free-floating thing it has been, and it also affected the amount of trust and openness that we had. It made things a little unsafe.

[Female, 35 years practice, 15 years in PSG]

I'm so happy when the person I don't like doesn't come.

[Female, 25 years practice, 20 years in PSG]

It was a real dilemma for me, because I didn't want to quit the group but I couldn't stand one of the other members, one of the founding members, in whose office we usually met. But I couldn't figure out how to address it. She was so narcissistic and so angry at her patients when they wouldn't do what she wanted, or wouldn't get better according to her schedule. I tried gently suggesting to her that she was angry at them, but she couldn't see it at all. I was about to quit when she announced that *she* was leaving to do training elsewhere. I was very relieved, because I really didn't want to quit the group.

[Male, 30 years practice, 25 years in PSG]

The woman who left was not someone I felt comfortable with. It was her way of intervening, her way of speaking. Not that she wasn't very bright, but there was something about her, that she would be the one to say something in a way that would be injurious, and not allow the group to work it through. Everyone else is comfortable with processing our own stuff. Even the way she left the group was arrogant, as if something about the rest of us didn't suit her.

[Female, 25 years practice, 1 year in PSG]

One woman denied disliking the other person but had difficulty dealing with her own reactions.

It's not that I don't like them, it's that I have to tiptoe around them, because I have to watch their fragility. I don't feel I can just be myself.

[Female, 25 years practice, 8 years in PSG]

## My own experience
There was, many years ago, someone in the group that I just didn't like. Something about the person just grated every time they said anything. It made being in the group difficult and often unpleasant, and I considered leaving and finding another group. But I stayed, and that person left the group before me. I'm glad I stuck it out. I wish I had been confident enough to confront the situation directly. I thought I was the only one feeling that way, and I was the newcomer. I assumed that others would have said something if they shared my feelings. It was only later on that I discovered there were other group members who did agree with me, but they also had said nothing.

This is yet another reason to be open and honest about what we are thinking and feeling about the group. If everyone had spoken up, maybe we would have been able to process and resolve some of the issues. Maybe we would both have remained in the group, and of us would have grown from the experience.

## Do group members refer patients to each other?

We all have to make referrals from time to time. A patient asks for a rec-ommendation for a family member, or a friend. Perhaps we don't have an open hour and want to send the patient to someone else. A group that knows each other well could easily function as a good source of referrals. When making a referral we want to be sure that the professional we refer to will do a good job. After years in a peer supervision group together, members come to know each other well, and so can trust the referral they make to be in good hands.

> I do refer to the other group members if I think the person will be a good fit for the client that I am referring to them.
> [Female, 5 years practice, 1 year in PSG]

> I do refer to other group members and appreciate receiving referrals. I am also glad to have a group of people that I trust to take referrals.
> [Female, 20 years practice, 12 years in PSG]

Almost everyone (with only two exceptions) said that group members refer patients to each other, although a few (three of those) also added that it didn't happen a lot. Several people mentioned that they were un-happy with the number of referrals coming to them from the group and wondered why group members were referring to other people in the group and not to them. Two people offered a possible explanation.

> I have had some problem at times feeling that people were not referring to me with the same frequency that I either refer to them or that they re-fer to each other. In the past year or so I believe that nobody has an excess of patients, and that there are not so many referrals flowing in any direction.
> [Female, 40 years practice, 17 years in PSG]

> I didn't have a lot of referrals to make, and I suspect people were refer-ring to people who would refer back.
> [Female, 40 years practice, 15 years in PSG]

Another person described some of the complications that may underlie a referral.

> I refer a lot of my students to the other members, and so we struggle with finding the right boundary for how much I'm going to share with them, how much they're going to share with me. Recently I referred a couple. I referred the guy to one person in the group, the couple to another, and the woman to the third person. The woman never called but the couple did go in. We talked about them in the group but the person who was seeing the man said it was too much information for her and so we stopped talking about them in the group.
>
> [Female, 20 years practice, 7 years in PSG]

## My own experience

The people in peer group with me are the clinicians whose work I know best. Normally, we would be referring patients to each other all the time. The state of the economy has brought the steady stream of patient referrals down to a trickle. Most of my referrals these days come from current and former patients.

I like knowing who I'm referring to. Some therapists make a better fit with a particular patient than others, because they are more knowledgeable about a particular situation or problem, or because their personal style fits better with that patient.

# Is there anyone you wouldn't refer to? Why not?

In many groups, members are confident in their colleagues and refer patients freely to all the other members of the group. But in fact only eight people said there was no one in their group to whom they would hesitate to refer a patient. Most professionals find themselves in a peer group with at least some members that they have doubts about, and would be hesitant to give referrals.

Sometimes the reason is an issue of competence, training, or ability.

> Some of the people are just beginning, and I would not refer to them yet.
>
> [Male, 40 years practice, 7 years in PSG]

> I had some concerns about what I saw as a clinical weakness.
>
> [Female, 40 years practice, 15 years in PSG]

> There's one person who is more of a professor than a practitioner.
>
> [Female, 10 years practice, 6 years in PSG]

I would not refer sexual problems to one man. He seems to lack the training and may be afraid to ask the questions necessary.

[Female, 20 years practice, 15 years in PSG]

Incompetence, concrete thinking, lack of professional commitment, lack of understanding. I lack trust in their ability to do the work.

[Female, 25 years practice, 20 years in PSG]

More often, though, the reservations about making a referral come out of a personal issue or problem.

I thought that she, personally, was too anxious and did not have good control of herself.

[Female, 35 years practice, 15 years in PSG]

The person is too direct, the quality of consistent holding warmth is missing.

[Male, 40 years practice, 15 years in PSG]

There's one person who is more of a professor than a practitioner.

[Female, 10 years practice, 6 years in PSG]

If somebody has narcissistic issues, and I think they get in the way of their ability to be flexible and work with people, then I become very cautious about referring to them.

[Female, 35 years practice, 2 years in PSG]

I wouldn't refer to the psychiatrist for psychotherapy, but I just referred someone to him for pharmacology. The obsessiveness that makes him less effective as a therapist would be very helpful.

[Male, 15 years practice, 1 year in PSG]

I have trouble with a couple of people, in terms of how they work with patients, and feel that their anxiety greatly impedes their process at times.

[Female, 40 years practice, 17 years in PSG]

I think upon occasion they could be too personal with their patients, reveal too much about themselves. Sometimes I think their judgment is off.

[Female, 30 years practice, 30 years in PSG]

I don't find them stable enough.

[Female, 40 years practice, 18 years in PSG]

It's hard to imagine him being a good therapist. He talks so much I think it would undermine therapy. The amount of talking he does would be really disturbing to me as a patient, so I don't want to subject someone to that.

[Male, 10 years practice, 3 years in PSG]

With two people, knowing things about them personally has really influenced whether I'd want to refer to them privately.

[Female, 25 years practice, 8 years in PSG]

They are maddeningly concrete.

[Male, 15 years practice, 5 years in PSG]

**My own experience**
I try to be careful about referrals. I believe I owe that to the prospective patient. There is a wide array of personalities and clinical styles in my group, and I try to make a good fit. Of course, I'm not limited in making referrals to only those people in the peer group. I can draw from several other professional groups that I belong to. If I thought it was the right fit, I would refer to everyone in my group.

# Has there ever been a crisis that threatened the existence of the group?

Occasionally something occurs in the group that is so serious that the very existence of the group is in question. Some groups survive these crises and some don't. Twenty-four people said there had been no such crisis; ten people said there had. Of these ten, four said their group had ended. Groups that face the issues directly are more likely to survive than those that don't address the group process itself, or those that do it reluctantly.

Several groups had to deal with a specific crisis situation.

I felt that the man who died was one of the linchpins of the group, and when he died, and the group didn't process that, and people didn't show up, I worried that the group might fall apart at that point. I thought, "Are people going to deal with this by not talking about it? Is this group going to become something I'm less invested in?" I was very angry at the people who made a choice not to come to group after the funeral. Some people had legitimate reasons but some people just chose not to come. I felt, "That's not right. What about us? We need them to be here." And that didn't feel so good. It felt kind of selfish.

[Female, 40 years practice, 17 years in PSG]

Early on, someone breached confidentiality. We dealt with it within the group. We didn't ask them to leave but the person left the group.
[Male, 45 years practice, 20 years in PSG]

Some groups end due to attrition, although the departures themselves may actually be due to a deeper problem that has been unaddressed or unresolved.

The group ended because of diminishing attendance, which was a result of the loss of administrative support in the clinic.
[Female, 30 years practice, 3 years in PSG]

One of the members had a family crisis, so he started not coming, and then that, even though it wasn't intentional, gave everyone, when they had their own mini-life crises, permission to bail out on the group.
[Female, 5 years practice, 1 year in PSG]

The group ended because people left. One left because he closed his practice to do organizational work. The four continued meeting for some time. Then another man said he was beginning analytic training and wouldn't have the time. That left three, and we tried meeting for a while but one of us also was doing a lot of other kinds of work and so we decided to end the group. We cast about for some new people but couldn't find anyone local.
[Female, 40 years practice, 15 years in PSG]

One of the remaining members may be leaving the area and the group, which would mean we're down to three.
[Female, 35 years practice, 32 years in PSG]

Some groups had to deal with a troublesome member.

There was someone who the group had a problem with. She couldn't hear what was going on, and she couldn't contain herself, which was very frustrating to the people who were presenting, and to the rest of us, because we couldn't get a word in edgewise. What we actually had to do, because she wasn't leaving, is end the group, and then reconstitute it, which was terrible. It was really hard. It took a year and a half. You don't want to do that to anyone and it took a really long time. We never felt that the group would totally disintegrate, but it did in a sense because it threatened the existence of the group as it was.
[Female, 35 years practice, 15 years in PSG]

A few people were anticipating the problems a diminishing membership can cause.

One person is leaving soon, and I'm thinking about leaving too, so we'll see how the group continues after that.
[Male, 15 years practice, 5 years in PSG]

It's hard that we only have four people, and one of us has moved away from the city and only comes in for the group every other meeting.
[Female, 35 years practice, 30 years in PSG]

Several people mentioned that they sometimes thought that there was a threat to the group when members were absent, or were in direct and overt conflict.

Sometimes I get worried that the group is breaking up when several people are missing. But I've asked a few people and they didn't have that feeling.
[Female, 30 years practice, 8 months in PSG]

When there's an argument I become nervous about that, but it's my own fear and there's never any real danger of that happening.
[Female, 40 years practice, 18 years in PSG]

**My own experience**
My first peer group, which ended after a year, died because too many people left. There was no specific crisis. I left the second group, but I think that group continued to meet. The current group has seen its share of conflicts, and of losses, but there has never been a situation that I would call a crisis, a moment in which the viability of the group itself was in question. I can't imagine anything that would so threaten the group that it would stop functioning. Because it has already survived thirty years and more, I think of it as unbreakable.

# What do you like best about the group?

There were many answers shading into other answers, so this question is hard to quantify. Many people mentioned the feeling of being supported by a community of colleagues in a safe space as the most important feature. Some people cited the holding environment, feeling accepted and validated. Others put these first: the friendship, the caring, the safety, the opportunity to get and give help; the intellectual stimulation, the variety of points of view.

A sense of being in a community of people who understand the work was very important to many people.

Most weeks there's nothing that I need to talk about. But I like the knowledge that every week in my practice I have, if something comes up and I've got a problem, I'm not going to have to wait more than a couple of days to deal with it, with a bunch of really smart, really experienced people. I have confidence that whatever it is that I can't think of, somebody will.

[Female, 25 years practice, 15 years in PSG]

I like the consistency of the support around the challenges of this profession. What's been particularly helpful to me in terms of my own issues is that the group has this mix of more academic and intellectually ambitious and accomplished people, with others who are not that prominent in the profession. I've always been conflicted about that issue: Am I good enough? Have I published enough? And in this group I'm sitting with people who have various views about that. It's very nice to feel so accepted being who I am.

[Male, 40 years practice, 15 years in PSG]

I like the support, the feeling of being a respected colleague in a community of professionals, and the security of having somewhere to bring the problems we all inevitably encounter.

[Male, 30 years practice, 25 years in PSG]

It's a solid group of friends, of colleagues, of community, that's there for me and I can count on and trust and safely open myself up to when I need to.

[Female, 30 years practice, 30 years in PSG]

It's a place that I need in order to talk about the cases that I'm working with and have metabolized all month. I've come to rely on that space the group offers me.

[Male, 15 years practice, 5 years in PSG]

I really like having that place to let my hair down. Not to be sitting alone with it.

[Female, 25 years practice, 1 year in PSG]

The sense of community contributes to the feeling of safety.

I like the people a lot. I have a lot of respect for them. I feel like, as a group, although we all work somewhat differently, we have a lot of respect for differences in how people work. I'm always glad to see people walk in.

[Female, 40 years practice, 17 years in PSG]

There's a sense of safety that we all have. We've all felt free enough to burst into tears or to talk about the way something's bringing up stuff from our own personal lives. We know a fair amount about each other at this point. It's a very non-shaming group.

[Female, 25 years practice, 11 years in PSG]

The warm, sometimes loving relationships with the other people create a personal, as well as professional, support network.

For all my impatience and wish for us to get down to business, I like the conviviality. It feels very warm. I always want to go. I really look forward to it.

[Female, 25 years practice, 15 years in PSG]

We really all care about each other.

[Female, 25 years practice, 8 years in PSG]

I like the fact that we feel connected to each other, and that we can call on each other for help, and it's something we can depend on.

[Female, 30 years practice, 8 months in PSG]

Seeing people I like, and seeing with what integrity they function.

[Male, 15 years practice, 1 year in PSG]

I love that I can talk about anything. It's very safe. I was diagnosed with cancer some years ago, and I could talk about what I was going through and how it was affecting the work, how I used work to distract myself from it, how it was important to me to feel in control because I couldn't control the illness. And now I have another medical issue, it's been the same. They'll cover for me while I'm in the hospital and at home.

[Female, 20 years practice, 15 years in PSG]

It's a warm, loving group. We really care for each other. I really feel good in it. I look forward to it and I feel safe in it.

[Female, 20 years practice, 7 years in PSG]

I like the feeling of community. I'm not that outgoing, and I like seeing those people that I knew and brought into the group.

[Female, 35 years practice, 30 years in PSG]

There's a forum where I can go. I'm never alone with my patients—or my life problems. It's wonderful. A couple of years ago when my husband was in the hospital and I thought I was going to lose him, I was on my way from my office to the hospital. The group was meeting, and I didn't think I could stay, but I stopped in, and I got so much support

just from knowing the group was here. We're like a very good family—
better than the real family.

> [Female, 45 years practice, 30 years in PSG]

Some people liked the intellectual aspects of the group.

I love the intellectual stimulation of it, and the collegiate support of
feeling like I'm not alone in my office.

> [Female, 5 years practice, 1 year in PSG]

I do sometimes get feedback that's very helpful.

> [Female, 25 years practice, 20 years in PSG]

I enjoy the level of competence. I come away being reinforced in my
theoretical orientation. It's a very good training.

> [Female, 35 years practice, 5 years in PSG]

As much as the different points of view can be confusing, I really enjoy
the variety. There are people who are very psychoanalytically trained,
very cognitively trained, a couple of psychiatrists with a lot of information about medication. There are a lot of different points of view.

> [Male, 10 years practice, 3 years in PSG]

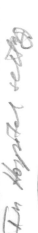

The opportunity to get help with difficult situations and to give help to
others was also important to a few people.

It's a forum for me to contribute and help other therapists work through
some issues with patients, and a place for me to do that too.

> [Male, 40 years practice, 8 months in PSG]

For one person, who worked in a hospital setting, the group was a special
experience.

It was probably the first time in all the years here that we actually had
time set aside for us to get together as peers to support and help each
other out.

> [Female, 30 years practice, 3 years in PSG]

## My own experience

One of the best parts of doing this book was getting to hear how happy
and excited some people are by the experience in their peer group. One
of the reasons I chose this topic is that I know that peer group can be
such an important part of one's professional career, and the people in the
group part of one's professional family, for life. I know this because it
has been that for me for so long.

## What do you like least about the group?

Even when people love their groups, there is usually some aspect they don't like so much. The most common complaint (nine people) was that there was a lack of focus, or of structure, in some area of the functioning of the group.

> There are times when we don't work with the clinical stuff we're carrying. The personal stuff preempts.
>
> [Male, 40 years practice, 15 years in PSG]

> There is a responsibility when you present to put your case together, and there is one group member who presents frequently and her cases are very disjointed and hard to follow, and it's hard to know what the issue is, and then I get resentful.
>
> [Female, 20 years practice, 12 years in PSG]

> Sometimes it's frustrating when people are off on their own tangent.
>
> [Female, 45 years practice, 30 years in PSG]

> I hate when someone monopolizes in an unfair way.
>
> [Female, 30 years practice, 30 years in PSG]

> I don't like the issue of getting down to work slower than I would want.
>
> [Female, 26 years practice, 1 year in PSG]

> All the other members are involved with an institute that I'm not part of, and I have limited tolerance for talk about the institute. It's like family gossip, but I'm not in that family, so who cares?
>
> [Female, 35 years practice, 5 years in PSG]

> Sometimes we get into too much chitchat.
>
> [Female, 20 years practice, 12 years in PSG]

> Sometimes I think that we don't do as much as we could. My past experience with these groups has involved more structure, for example, reading articles and presenting. When I worked in the agency we did live family work, with a team behind the mirror. I miss that level of sophistication.
>
> [Female, 20 years practice, 15 years in PSG]

Seven people had problems with the time commitment or travel requirements of regular attendance.

Sometimes it feels like pressure to be here. I'm in another group that meets once a month, and sometimes it conflicts. When I'm here I like to come to group but I often have something else I'm doing.

[Female, 35 years practice, 30 years in PSG]

It's hard to get here sometimes, because I live so far away.

[Male, 40 years practice, 8 months in PSG]

I hate having to physically show up when I'm tired.

[Male, 15 years practice, 1 year in PSG]

Sometimes there's something I would rather do with that time, because I don't have a problem to discuss. But I have a commitment to the group and I show up.

[Female, 25 years practice, 15 years in PSG]

Three people thought that there were not enough different points of view, and one person from a very large group thought there were too many.

We're talking about adding another person. It would be nice to get more perspectives.

[Female, 35 years practice, 15 years in PSG]

There aren't enough people in the group who run groups.

[Male, 15 years practice, 5 years in PSG]

We all know each other so well that I think we might be missing something.

[Female, 25 years practice, 11 years in PSG]

Sometimes there are too many points of view.

[Male, 10 years practice, 3 years in PSG]

Three people said there was not enough time, or the group met too infrequently.

There have been times where I didn't bring something up because other people had something urgent, and after the meeting I wished I had brought it up. As I measured their urgency, mine didn't seem that urgent, and yet when they talked about whatever they talked about, mine seemed just as urgent, but I didn't define it that way. The issue is competing for time.

[Female, 40 years practice, 17 years in PSG]

I don't like the fact that we meet only once a month.

[Male, 40 years practice, 7 years in PSG]

I don't like that we meet so infrequently. I'd like more time to talk and present and share problems. I also think if we met more frequently we'd have to deal with process more, which I think would lead to our development as better group therapists. It would be a more intense learning environment.

[Female, 35 years practice, 2 years in PSG]

Three people said there was insufficient processing of the group itself.

The failure to process what happens in the room is a real issue for me. Some of the group members really don't deal with their feelings very well. They're really unable to sit with their feelings and become very defensive.

[Female, 24 years practice, 20 years in PSG]

This group isn't interested in looking at group process within the group. We do it only when we have to, like when two people are fighting or recently when a member left unexpectedly. I wish we did it more regularly.

[Male, 30 years practice, 25 years in PSG]

Two people mentioned a lack of commitment, often manifested as a lack of attendance.

I don't like the lack of commitment and accountability.

[Female, 5 years practice, 1 year in PSG]

I hate when people don't show up.

[Female, 30 years practice, 8 months in PSG]

Two people said that they had a conflict with another group member.

I hate the occasions when I don't feel safe, when this other member will take that superior view and I feel trumped.

[Female, 20 years practice, 7 years in PSG]

I really don't like the tension with the other woman.

[Female, 40 years practice, 15 years in PSG]

Two people had a problem with the referrals made within the group.

Some of my own unresolved stuff comes up in terms of people being friendly with each other. Why aren't they as friendly with *me*? Why didn't they ask *me* to have lunch with them today? I get competitive in friendships, and feeling left out. And sometimes when people are talk-

ing about a patient they have in common, I think, "How come they
didn't refer this patient to *me*?"

> [Female, 40 years practice, 17 years in PSG]

I don't like that they don't refer enough people to me.

> [Female, 30 years practice, 18 years in PSG]

Two people who were from very small groups wished the group were
larger.

> I wish there were more people.
>
> [Male, 45 years practice, 20 years in PSG]

One person said that the group was not honest enough in their feedback.

> When I came into the group, I found that everyone was just making
> nice with each other. I said I was very uncomfortable because there's
> no confrontation, no reactions. It seemed unreal.
>
> [Male, 45 years practice, 5 years in PSG]

Only four people said there was nothing they could think of that they
didn't like.

> I'd have to make something up, like washing the dishes after they
> leave. It's on Fridays and sometimes I'd like to get out of town early,
> but I don't because I think it's important.
>
> [Female, 35 years practice, 30 years in PSG]

## My own experience
Sometimes I wish I had the day to myself. Sometimes the group seems
diffuse and unfocused, and the presentations scattered or unchallenging.
Sometimes I'm tired or distracted and can't pay attention. All of these
are rare, and are usually not a reaction to the group itself, but of where I
find myself that day.

# Have you ever thought about leaving the group?

The majority of the interviewees (twenty-two) said they never even think
about leaving the group. Another nine said they at least occasionally
think about it; four of them seriously consider leaving or are already
planning to leave. The remaining three said that their groups had already
ended.

These people are considering leaving their groups.

> A couple of people had already decided that they wanted a different group. I'm actually thinking of forming a new group with some of the members of this group. There are other people leaving at the same time I am.
>
> [Female, 25 years practice, 20 years in PSG]

> I told them, when the woman who drives me crazy wasn't there, that I was very unhappy with the group.
>
> [Male, 45 years practice, 5 years in PSG]

Sometimes people are unsure that the group they are in is the right one for them.

> I sometimes feel that I could be learning more somewhere else. But then I think that while that might be true, I would be losing the safety of this group, which is hard to find.
>
> [Female, 25 years practice, 11 years in PSG]

> I'm not sure if it's the best group for me. Also, when I'm very busy, I question the value.
>
> [Male, 10 years practice, 3 years in PSG]

> I've thought about it a few times, but I've never allowed myself to. I thought the group was different from me, a different mentality. I've never left because I've been aware that my feelings might not be objective.
>
> [Female, 40 years practice, 18 years in PSG]

> The thought crosses my mind from time to time but I don't give it much weight. I wonder if there might be a group I'm better suited to.
>
> [Male, 30 years practice, 25 years in PSG]

> I have because only one other person does group therapy and I want to be able to talk about my groups. I'm also thinking of leaving because the person who brought me in is leaving soon. Plus it's far away and takes an hour there and an hour back in addition to the group itself.
>
> [Male, 15 years practice, 5 years in PSG]

Time commitment is often an issue.

> I have so little free time that I resent having to get up and go on a day when I don't see patients. I guard my time jealously but I guess it's worth it.
>
> [Female, 10 years practice, 6 years in PSG]

I hate having to physically show up when I'm tired. For that reason only, I think about it.

[Male, 15 years practice, 1 year in PSG]

There was a point where I wanted to get into a leader-led group, or take
a course, and I would need to stop coming to the group during those
months that the course is given.

[Female, 35 years practice, 30 years in PSG]

Even when a group ends people often try to find peer supervision somehow.

I still do peer supervision with two different individuals on a consistent
basis. I meet with one in particular for lunch every week, and we speak
often during the week. It feels more accountable and more reliable and
consistent and necessary. I do miss the other people's perspectives, and
also the actual meeting of a group.

[Female, 5 years practice, 1 year in PSG]

When the group works well, people are happy to continue. It is for many
peer group members an important component of their professional lives.

I see it going on forever.

[Female, 35 years practice, 15 years in PSG]

I don't know what people do without something like this.

[Female, 25 years practice, 15 years in PSG]

**My own experience**
The last comment above sums it up for me: I don't know how people in
private practice survive without a peer group. I've been in my group for
such a long time (most of us have lost exact count of how long we've
been there), and it's always been an essential and crucial part of my professional life, so much so that it's impossible to imagine not being in
such a group.

# Discussion

In the best functioning groups, members get so much—support, comfort, wisdom, insight, challenge, growth, validation, and camaraderie—it
may have been hard to narrow it down to one or two things. On the other
hand, nothing is perfect, and we would expect that something about
every group would be objectionable to someone. On balance, most

people like being in their groups; some people love it. I don't think it means too much that there is an aspect one doesn't like if one likes the rest well enough.

Conflict is an area where the group really has to address things directly. Even then the situation may not be fixable. Sometimes people are in the wrong group, and they need to find another one. Too many groups avoid dealing directly with the problems, and sometimes the group falls apart under the weight of unaddressed issues.

I am quite certain that the biggest threat to a group's existence is the failure to address and process difficult feelings about the group itself. Members carrying a lot of hurt, resentment, or frustration tend to miss meetings, which can give other members a tacit permission to also be absent, and the group can disintegrate. Most groups die slowly, not all at once, and timely intervention can sometimes revive a dying group. Sometimes a crisis can be useful, because it can alert everyone that there are unaddressed issues, and give the group an opportunity to finally address them.

Some disagreement is inevitable: members are different and will react in individual ways in the same situation. Occasionally two people have such different styles and ways of working, or even thinking about the work, that they regularly clash with each other about what to do or how to do it. In a well-functioning group, there is room for this, and eventually the two will likely stop butting heads and accept the differences.

In peer group, we find ourselves in intimate connection with a variety of people, some of whom we did not choose. It's hard to acknowledge a personal dislike for another group member. It can seem almost like a failure on the part of the disliker, more than on the part of the dislikee. Another person can push old buttons, not unlike the way a patient can. Again, I think a well-functioning group can tolerate a certain amount of this tension, especially if it is out on the table and being discussed.

On the other hand, we must also recognize that groups differ from each other in many ways, and if a member is continually dissatisfied or unhappy, then he or she might be in the wrong group. I would urge anyone dissatisfied with the way his or her group is functioning to bring that up and discuss the issue with the group. Sometimes the problem can be resolved. Sometimes it can't, and the person needs to find another group. If the group is unwilling or unable to deal with the member's dissatisfaction, that would be a very strong indication that this is not the right group.

We all, in the course of our training as therapists, had supervision from more experienced teachers. At some point in one's career, the time arrives to step up and take responsibility for oneself. I see peer group as analogous to adulthood: we don't need parents to instruct us or to teach us how to behave. It's empowering to let the group be in charge of itself and not to need an authority to arbitrate or direct.

I love the way a peer group manages itself. The members are responsible for structuring the group. When there are conflicts, people deal with them without needing a higher authority. I think that, after many years of training and experience, most clinicians have the tools they need to handle the situation themselves.

Peer groups can be one of the best resources for referrals. People get to know each other's work well, and can refer with some confidence about what kind of treatment the patient will get. Knowing other professionals from meetings and conferences doesn't always reveal who they are or how they actually work in their offices. In a large group, there are many therapists to choose from and one can tailor the referral to the patient.

It seems obvious that, in any group, one will prefer some practitioners to others in terms of style, personality, manner, theoretical orientation, and competence. Too often I have seen referrals made more on the basis of friendship than on professional ability. We have a responsibility to the patient to make sure we are making the best possible referral.

# Part III

# Some Groups

# Chapter 8

# Specific Peer Groups

There are, of course, some commonalities among all the peer supervision groups I encountered in the course of doing this book, as well as important differences. Some groups are very structured, some are very spontaneous. Some have three people, some have twelve. Some are all men, some all women. Some meet every week, some only once a month. The previous section addressed some specific questions and issues in peer groups. Now let's look at some specific groups.

## Group 1—Spontaneous Generation

This first group is a well-established one that has been meeting for twenty years. It began almost accidently when one member "went to a party and a couple of my colleagues were talking about how it would be a good idea to get together and have a place where we can talk." They added another person and that made them a group. There have been other members coming in and leaving, but the membership has been stable with these three for the past ten years.

The group is very freely organized; the only explicit contractual agreements are honesty and confidentiality. Early in the life of the group, there was a crisis when "someone breached confidentiality." The group survived but the individual didn't. "We didn't ask them to leave, but the person left the group."

This group talks about professional matters, but also covers whatever areas in their personal lives members choose to bring into the discussion. As in many groups, whoever feels the most urgency gets to speak first. People present whatever is troubling them, personal or professional.

Presenters look for "a different opinion," or to deal with "feeling stuck," or to explore having "any type of emotional reaction" to a patient.

173

As in the next group, they don't see each other socially outside of the group, and so they may feel more freedom to explore the personal aspects of professional practice.

This group has been extremely stable for such a small number of people, and members like "the openness, the friendliness, and the nonjudgmental atmosphere." The only thing missing is more people, although if they haven't added anyone in ten years that can't be accidental. They are careful when giving feedback not to criticize or shame, but they can be "confrontational at times," especially when someone "isn't acting in his or her best interest" and then they can "become *very* confrontational."

## Group 2—Practice Development

This group consists of three people, two women and one man, and is organized around the issues of practice development: how to build and maintain a caseload in a private office, "the hidden side of practice, the business part." Another way of describing the focus is "the intersection of clinical work with the business that we're trying to maintain." The group is intentionally small. "We want to grow organically from within, rather than casting a wide net and bringing in a lot of new people. We've all encountered people who've expressed interest in joining us, but we're still at the stage of exploring and discovering our rhythm and our way of working."

The group does not socialize with each other, and doesn't discuss their personal lives, although "it is inevitable, when you're talking about topics like money, that you're going to be talking about personal life." A lot of the discussion concerns fees, "fee setting, nonpayment," but they might also talk about an unexpected termination. A lot of time is given to discussing promotion and self-promotion, "how you market yourself."

Because this is a new group, only in existence for six months, people are still finding their way, feeling out the other members, exploring ways of speaking and giving feedback. "There's a certain degree of testing the waters, what can I feel free to speak about, what is allowed, what will I allow myself to say?" Because the group is small, people get to present every meeting and there is no competition for group time.

Having everyone focused on the same issues reveals a "universality, in that we're all faced with similar challenges." Members take comfort in knowing they have a forum to raise issues and ask questions about aspects of professional practice that many therapists avoid discussing.

# Group 3—A Group of Beginners

All the members of this group had been in training together and wanted to continue having a place to meet and discuss cases, "getting the peer support around our cases and being in private practice." This group started with one man and four women, and the women looked to the lone man to provide the male point of view. They met in the same office every other week for two hours.

The group decided that they wanted to be fairly structured, so they chose a format that allowed that they "would each spend twenty minutes talking about cases, and someone would be the timekeeper." They focused on family and couple therapy, since that had been their training. Because all were relatively new practitioners, members presented cases where they felt stuck, or where lack of knowledge or experience made it hard to get a handle on the case. They also presented situations that would provide "good learning opportunities" for everyone.

The group was sensitive to each other's feelings and was careful about how they gave feedback. Their training had taken a "strength" perspective, which focused on client strengths, not weaknesses, and they used this model in the group as well, focusing on therapist strengths and abilities, and being careful not to criticize. Because they were all new to private practice, however, they sometimes missed having an "expert to give us their lens of experience."

The group survived for only a year. Of the five members, two were often absent, which destabilized the group and made it easier for other members to miss meetings. "One of the members had a family crisis, so he started not coming, and then that gave everyone, when they had their own mini-life-crises, permission to bail out on the group." Undercurrents and issues were often not addressed. Overall, it was "a pretty passive group." There were several people in the group who "avoided conflict in general."

# Group 4—A Women's Group

This is a remarkably stable group of seven women that has been meeting for eight years, without anyone leaving or joining. It formed out of a group that met with a leader, which ended, and the group decided to continue meeting. Because of the members' training and orientation, the group focuses specifically on work with couples.

As in so many groups, there is no explicit contract other than confidentiality. In the old group, the leader provided the structure, and without a leader now there is much more crosstalk and interruption. The group has considered assigning someone the role of Keeper of the Space, whose job it is to "keep the space clear for the person who's talking." Some members find the crosstalk disturbing, even upsetting. The group can sometimes feel unfocused.

Some people have connections outside the group, and these sub-groups may interfere with the ongoing discussion. Some members come from out of town, and their absences are "detrimental to the cohesiveness of the group." In spite of the structural issues, members seem happy to be there.

This is the only group who suggested that they might hire an outside consultant to come into the group, and also the only group who said that members might bring in videotapes of their work for the group to look at and discuss. When conflict arises between two people, the group helps them resolve the issue by mirroring and mediating. Feedback can be di-rect, and, while not shaming, can make it clear that the group does not agree with or even approve of what the presenter has done with the pa-tient.

# Group 5—A Countertransference Group

This group of six members is unusually well balanced: three men and three women; two psychiatrists, two psychologists, two social workers. The different kinds of training and experience allow the group to provide "very different ways of conceptualizing what's going on," which they consider a real advantage. They've been meeting for sixteen years, every week for an hour and a half, which is more often than most of our groups. The group grew out of a previous peer group that had disbanded when several members moved their offices. That group had not had the cohesion of this one; it didn't always feel so helpful and, while "there was nothing wrong with it, it just wasn't compelling." People were added in the new location and a new group was formed, with only person leav-ing because "she didn't fit."

The group begins, as so many of our groups do, with some personal checking in, noting any situations in the members' personal lives that affect their state of mind, and therefore the work. If the situation is a ge-nuine crisis, a medical emergency, or an important personal loss, the group might spend the entire session discussing that. But normally, after a few minutes, they get down to business. They have an understanding that most of the time their topic and focus will be countertransference, "personal upsets and dilemmas with patients," and they used to think of themselves as "the countertransference group."

Clinical material can sometimes include gender issues, and then the group may find itself dividing along gender lines, the men's reactions contrasted with the women's. The group is careful with feedback, making sure to give comments in a "kindly and gentle way. There is a real sense of respect and safety." In spite of the careful thoughtfulness, "sometimes someone's been really injured, or feels misunderstood," and the group will process that until everyone feels resolved. But the group is clear that they are not a therapy group, and not a process group. "We are not there to interpret each other in any way." Some members might wish there was more opportunity to say directly to someone, "I think the way you talk about that, you have a problem with it."

The group has dealt with open conflict, when one of its members "felt judged, and complained about feeling unsupported, and announced one day that she wasn't coming anymore." The rest of the group thought that "it wasn't working for her. She didn't fit," and so they allowed her to leave without processing her complaints. Overall, the members of this group love being there and never think about leaving.

## Group 6—A Very Large Group

This group of twelve men meets monthly for two hours. The group is so large that it's rare for everyone to show up. The size of the group makes it possible to have a large enough group even when several people are missing. This large group contains many different individual points of view and theoretical orientations and, especially when everyone is in attendance, the feedback can be so varied as to be confusing. For some members, it's a relief when people are absent because the group seems a manageable size and the feedback isn't too confusing.

As with so many groups, there is no contract, and the only agreement is confidentiality. There are two members who function as informal leaders, and help structure the discussion. The group tries to cover two cases and one issue per meeting. Issues could be something like "ending the session on time, or what to do when your practice hours drop down, or handling cancellations."

The combination of large group size and infrequent meeting (once a month) puts time at a premium. Sometimes the agenda is set before the group by email. The group recognizes that presentations can ramble and get diffuse, so they limit the time allotted, and tell presenters to focus specifically on what they want from the group. But sometimes people present a new patient, and the discussion is less specific because "they just want to talk about someone they just started seeing and get some feedback."

All peer groups struggle with the problem of how to tell presenters that what they did with a patient was questionable. In this group, some members have had negative reactions in the past to the group's comments, feeling criticized and shamed. Now the group tries to manage feedback so that it feels supportive and useful, and so would not make members hesitate to bring in difficult cases.

## Group 7—A Group about Group

This group is composed entirely of group therapists, and limits most of the presentations and discussions to the difficulties and problems encountered running therapy groups. The six members, three men and three women, are all experienced group therapists, and meet once a month for an hour and a half. They acknowledge that it's not really often enough, but other schedule commitments make meeting more often impossible. For various reasons, someone is often absent. This interferes with group functioning, but creates some feelings that can be dealt with in the process part of the work.

The group was formed a year ago, when two people from another group that had recently disbanded wanted to continue meeting. Candidates were selected consciously and carefully to fit with the topic and the other members, and also because they seemed to be "capable of not just discussing cases from an intellectual perspective, but also had the capacity and openness to exploring things on a deeper level, including any dynamics that emerged in the group itself."

This group intentionally is a process group, believing that exploring the process in the group itself will illuminate the process in the groups they run in their practices. Members find "that if we're talking about the group process, someone is likely to bring it back to the groups that we're leading."

There are very few rules and no explicit contract. Often, someone simply starts talking about a problem, and it's up to the other members to say if they also need time to present. All the members are used to being in groups and used to leading groups, so the leadership functions are dispersed among the group. "It doesn't reside in any one person, which is a measure of a high-functioning peer group." When conflicts arise, as they sometimes do, the group helps the individuals address the feelings and discover the source of the conflict. "What makes for an effective group is the capacity of those two people to look at their own stuff." This is where a lot of experience in groups can help.

This group is unusual, at least among our somewhat limited sample, in the way it intentionally and regularly looks at the process of the group itself. Most groups do it reluctantly, with some trepidation and only when they absolutely must, to avoid major crisis and group dissolution. It's much harder to talk about something happening in the group in the moment than it is to describe a problem in one's private practice.

## Group 8—A Group in Trouble

This group of eight people, four men and four women, meets monthly for two hours. Meetings rotate among the homes and offices of the members. The group has been in existence over twenty years, and three of the founding members are still in the group. There have been losses of original members: two members died prematurely, and others moved away. The group hasn't adequately processed these deaths, and there is some unfinished mourning.

The existence of the group these days is a little precarious. People are often absent, especially if the weather is bad. Several people are unhappy with the way the group functions. Some feel that they can't get the help they need with specific situations because the other members aren't knowledgeable in those areas. Some members are disturbed by the lack of expertise in general. "Some people will bring up very mundane things that they really should know; it's rather astounding."

Others are unhappy that the group never seems to address the issues in the group itself, and little processing goes on. "Sometimes they're open to hearing it and experiencing it, and sometimes they aren't." Conflicts can go unaddressed, and unresolved. "Whatever conflict has arisen, nothing has come out of it." The group seems unaware of ways to process the issue. "There's a degree of resistance to discussing the process and dynamics in the group, or even a lack of awareness of those dynamics. Some of the group members really don't deal with their feelings very well. They're really unable to sit with their feelings and become very defensive."

Several of the members are so dissatisfied that they are planning to leave the group soon. This will destabilize the group, and it may not survive these losses.

# Group 9—A Deeper Look

Because this is my own peer supervision group, I was able to interview all nine members, and so will be able to examine in some detail the dynamics and functioning of the group.

The group was organized over thirty years ago. Some aspects of its beginnings are lost in the cloudy memories of the survivors. There were at least five members at the beginning; three still remain in the group. One founder left to pursue other interests; one died unexpectedly a year ago. Five other members have all been in the group between fifteen and twenty-five years. The one new person joined a little over a year ago. There have been others in the group, sometimes for years, sometimes only for a few months. Some left when their schedules no longer permitted them to attend meetings. A few left because they didn't fit with the others, and it was not the right group for them.

Half the group has been in other peer supervision groups in the past, all of which lasted a short while. Those groups did not come together the way this one has. They were too divergent or uncommitted. It is important to note that even though those groups did not survive, these members knew that they wanted the experience and kept seeking another group until they found one that worked. All the members want the support, collegiality, continued learning, and relief of professional isolation that peer supervision provides.

At the time of the interviews, there were seven women and two men in the group. Two are psychologists; five are social workers; two are psychoanalysts. This variety of backgrounds gives some range to group responses and reactions to member presentations. All members are experienced clinicians, with no one having less than twenty years experience, and a few having forty years and more. One person has a full-time agency position during the regular workweek, in addition to a smaller private practice; all the rest are exclusively in private practice. In addition to many years of practice, all members have had many years of personal therapy, and are knowledgeable about themselves and about the experience of being the patient.

The group meets every other week for an hour and a half, usually in the same office, unless that person is away and then the meeting moves to another location nearby. Most members practice in the same neighborhood; a few come from other areas. Food is not served, and normally people do not eat anything during the meeting. There are no fees or other financial obligations, although when flowers or other gifts are given on special occasions everyone chips in.

These people are friends as well as colleagues, and people often meet for lunch, movies, or theater. Almost everyone attends weddings, and other major celebrations. Members all seem to feel that they are connected in basic and important ways. Occasionally, when they hear about a social connection between other members, people may feel left out and wonder why they weren't included. No one feels that these social connections and contacts compromise the functioning of the group; many believe they enhance the commitment.

If there was ever a contract for the group, it hasn't been discussed since the beginning more than thirty years ago. Other than confidentiality, there are no explicit agreements. People are very careful about confidentiality, and patient's last names are never mentioned. If a member of the group knows the patient, then discussion of the case only happens if that member is absent.

In the past, there have been people in the group that were problematic for some of the other members. Their personalities grated, they didn't seem competent, or they appeared self-absorbed and uncaring about the others. But all these people have left the group years ago, and everyone likes all the current members.

Referrals are the lifeblood of anyone in private practice, and peer groups can be a great source of referrals. These are the colleagues who best know the style of work, and the level of ability, of the other members. In this group, people make referrals very consciously and carefully, although in the current economic climate there are few referrals to make.

The women in the group have always outnumbered the men, but no one describes any gender-based differences in the way people participate. The men are no more aggressive than the women, or less nurturing. Everyone notices differences among the members, but these are seen as determined by individual character, not gender. Some of the women think that the men might be more aggressive if there were more men, and the fact that the women so outnumber them keeps them in check. Others think that, because there are only two men, their words might carry more weight.

Most members believe that absences undermine the functioning of the group, but it's rare that anyone has been confronted about being absent. When everyone is present the room is very full, and someone will remark that it has been a long time since this has happened. The group is large enough that, even with several absences, there is still a group. But continuity gets ragged, and some people know more than others about the cases being presented. Confronting an issue in the group itself becomes much more difficult when people are missing.

The group has tried reading papers and books on certain topics related to whatever they might be discussing, but this has not lasted long. Some people want to include this reading as a regular part of the group, but more people are not interested and feel that it takes away from the time spent on clinical issues and cases, which is their first priority. Occasionally, someone has by force of personality gotten the group to read something, but it happens less than once a year.

Although some people feel occasionally unsafe without a designated leader, most like the equality of being peers; it feels more grown up. Most of the members see themselves as experienced enough to lead a group themselves, and don't want to defer to anyone else's leadership, or put themselves back in a role that feels a little infantilized. They are happy that leadership functions are distributed among the members, and that no one is competing for the leader's attention or approval. Some people saw the recently deceased founding member as a kind of de facto leader, a father figure who could calm the waters and reassure the group that everything would be all right. His comforting presence is sometimes missed, especially in moments of conflict or other turmoil.

As people trickle in, they converse about more personal things with whoever is there. They report major events, and might announce the need for time to discuss a case. In general, there is some social chat and catching up at the beginning of each meeting. Some people feel this often goes on too long. Meeting time is allotted when everyone has arrived and the group can assess how many people need time, and how much they need. A presenter will often know that his or her question will be quickly answered. Other presentations will go into more depth and take more time. There may sometimes be competition for the limited time that the group meets. Occasionally, people are conflicted about how urgently they need to discuss their case, and might defer to others, only to regret it later on.

The presenter will review the case, giving patient history and the history of the treatment. Sometimes the other members feel inundated by facts, and aren't clear about what the presenter needs, or what the question is exactly. At times it feels to some that the discussion is being monopolized, and one person is unfairly dominating the group, but this is rarely expressed. Members ask questions and give feedback—"Here's what comes up for me when I listen to this case." The presenter says when he or she has gotten what was needed, and the next presenter starts.

Normally, two or three cases are covered in the ninety minutes, and occasionally a few small issues as well.

Everyone understands that, if the case was going along well, they probably wouldn't be hearing about it in the group. The group is careful about giving feedback, trying hard not to criticize or shame. Sometimes a presenter reports feeling those things nevertheless, and the group tries to look at how that happened. Overall, people feel safe enough in the group to report even those situations they are least proud of, the ones that push all the personal buttons, even the ones where the presenter knows he or she hasn't done the best work. All group members are experienced enough and confident enough in their professionalism to tolerate hearing that they were stuck in a personal countertransference reaction, or missed something important, or misunderstood something about the patient.

People who present one week will usually report back the following meeting on what happened in the next session with the patient, and how the feedback from the group has impacted the treatment. Usually, there has been a positive effect, and the logjam is broken so that things can flow again. Sometimes the presenter realizes that the patient is psychologically less developed than he or she appeared, and the therapist can back up and slow down and expect less, which can take pressure off both the therapist and the patient.

Over the years there have been occasional conflicts. Although this scares some of the people, no one thinks that the existence of the group has ever actually been in danger. Some of the members have struggled with angry feelings toward each other. They sometimes feel disrespected and misunderstood. These angry feelings have flared up occasionally, and when that has happened someone else has stepped in to moderate and mediate the discussion. Other times one person or another has felt interrupted, or not listened to, dismissed, discounted. The tension in the room gets heavier, but the dispute has always been dealt with and resolved.

Many years ago, there was someone in the group who was difficult for many of the other members. They found that person self-absorbed and unable to hear feedback from the other members of the group. At least one new person who came into the group left soon after in reaction to that specific individual and the tension in the room. Some members, while unhappy about the situation, accepted it and said nothing. Others thought about leaving, but didn't want to lose their places in the group. It was only when that individual left to pursue other training that negative feelings emerged for discussion by the rest of the group.

The group has never given much attention to process, discussing what is happening in the group itself. Some members remind the others that it is not a therapy group, and some issues go unaddressed, or get cursory attention. Some members of the group seem to think that it might be too fragile to tolerate this kind of interaction, but others believe that addressing group process can only strengthen the connection and solidify the group even more.

In spite of the complaints and areas of dissatisfaction, group members are overall very satisfied with the group and no one talks about quitting. For most, leaving is unimaginable, and they picture themselves staying in this group forever.


## Discussion

We can see from even this small array that there are many different ways of being a peer group. Groups can assemble around concrete issues, like practice building, or themes, like countertransference, or social networks, such as those groups that form because the members all happen to have trained together, or just happen to be friends. All are equally valid ways of organizing.

Each can provide different strengths, and can address the members' feelings of needing help in a specific area. There is limited time in any group, and focusing on a particular aspect of the work may be how the members want to spend that time.

I personally prefer a group without a specific theme, in which anything can be the focus of the discussion. Of course, most groups will allow this, but perhaps some members, especially people new to the group, might hesitate to bring up those issues that seem "off topic." I think it is likely that, over time, groups that begin with a particular theme or topic expand to think of themselves as more inclusive of all the problems that arise in being a therapist.

We can see from some of these descriptions that being in a group is not automatically a source of happiness and relief. Some groups don't function very well, and even in those that do people may be unhappy with some aspect of group life. In the best functioning groups, there will be a mechanism for discussion of those dissatisfactions, and maybe the problem will be solved. But maybe not, and the person will have to reexamine whether this is the place to be, or if some other group would be a better fit.

I think that too often people leave a group without bringing up their problems with the group's functioning. I have seen this in my own group, where people have left with an explanation that seemed questionable to the rest of us. I wish they had revealed what the real issue was—maybe we could have addressed and even repaired it.

At best, a well-running peer group is like the good family that so many of us never had. We can reveal ourselves without fear or ridicule or punishment. We feel supported in our professional dreams and aspirations. We feel understood and accepted as we are. We feel safe. These qualities are not to be lightly dismissed or undervalued.

On the other side of the coin, dysfunctional groups can replicate our less-than-ideal families of origin. We can feel unfairly or hurtfully criticized. We can be shamed or humiliated. We can feel unsafe. Even in this situation, we are no longer helpless children, and we can speak up and address the problems. Maybe they can be repaired. If not, we are free to leave, something children can't do, and find another family.

I have made it clear that I believe strongly that every independent practitioner ought to be in a peer supervision group. In the next section, I present some guidelines for creating a group, or improving one that is not functioning well.

We have Clinical / professional +

<u>Not therapy</u>:

Do we want / need
Can we form our own
peer group ?

Our
(Purpose
or Task)  :  add /
more Clinical

# Conclusions and Recommendations

For me, this quote from one of the interviews is the essence of peer group: "We wanted a place to talk about some difficulties with cases that we all had. We were all very experienced, and didn't feel like we needed a supervisor, but that we could all be each other's supervisors." I wish every clinician could have this experience for at least some time, if not for life.

We have seen the advantages and potential drawbacks of being in a peer supervision group. Here are some of my own guidelines and recommendations for optimizing the experience.

## Purpose

Goldberg (1981) suggests that there are four primary reasons practitioners seek out peer supervision. The first purpose (clinical) is to have somewhere to bring difficult cases, issues, and situations. The second (professional) is that the peer group can become an important source of patient referrals. The third (emotional) is that the group provides support, encouragement, and validation. The last reason (social) is that the group can provide an antidote to the professional isolation of private practice. I think these are all good reasons to want to join a peer group, and while the first reason, discussing clinical problems and difficulties, may be paramount, all are valid reasons for joining.

Counselman and Weber (1994) call this central purpose of group function the *task*, and in this situation the task would be consultation and feedback. They point out that, in this setting, members will often have to discuss their countertransference reactions, and that this kind of "sharing personal material in a consultation group can be exciting and enrich the group but is a slippery slope in terms of task" (p. 353).

Both Goldberg and Counselman and Weber seem to fear that the temptation to turn the peer group into a therapy group will somehow prevail, and that the original purpose will be lost. I don't think this is a rea-

187

listic concern. In almost thirty years in three different groups, I never encountered anyone who ever suggested it, or came anywhere near acting as if it were desirable.

## Group size

In doing this book, I encountered groups of anywhere from three to twelve people. Three seems too small to me for several reasons. Even one absence makes it less than a group, and there are not enough different points of view to offer a presenter new takes on a case. On the other side, twelve seems too large, unless several people are always going to miss the meeting. There may be too much competition for group time, and so many opinions may be confusing. I think anywhere from five to ten people would be optimal size, although any size group is better than none at all.

## Membership / Composition

It is important to have at least some experienced clinicians in the group. It might be possible to have some less experienced members as well, because it would be great for them to learn from their elders, but the danger of that arrangement is that they might find presenting their work, with all its mistakes and rough edges, too shaming. So it might work better if all members are at roughly the same point in their careers, which implies that they are also in the same age range.

While some of the people who participated come from groups that are all men or all women, most of them acknowledged that something is missing as a result. I think both male and female points of view are complementary and necessary for fully understanding any patient.

Goldberg (1981) suggests that members should have sufficient personal therapy so that their personal issues don't interfere with their functioning in the group. Obviously, someone who has dealt with his or her personal issues in treatment is less likely to have them triggered by a patient or by another member of the peer group. Most experienced clinicians have had a lot of therapy, both individual and group, and understand the value of the process of looking at themselves. I don't see how trying to keep out of the group anyone who hasn't had sufficient personal therapy is going to work. No matter how much therapy one has had, there is always the possibility that some old button will be pushed. A well-functioning group will be able to handle this when it occurs.

## Frequency and Time

The groups in this book met weekly, biweekly, and monthly. The first two make sense to me; monthly seems too infrequent. A problem in treatment may not keep for several weeks. It would be hard to wait that long before being able to consult with the group.

I think an hour and a half is the minimum time for a productive meeting, and it could easily be two hours and longer. Some groups try to make up for infrequent meetings with extended session times, but I don't think that's an effective solution, because there is still too long between meetings to be able to respond to immediate needs, and because continuity is going to be difficult.

## Location

It doesn't matter whether the group meets in the same place all the time or rotates among the members' spaces, or whether the meetings take place in homes or offices. Whatever feels fair and practical to the membership will work. I don't think it makes sense to try to hold a meeting in a public space, like a restaurant. Confidentiality could be compromised, and the discussion would be inhibited.

## Fees

Most groups had no financial contribution as part of their commitment. One group collected funds for a very specific purpose: promoting the group as a referral source. One interviewee thought that not paying for the group was a factor in its failure to survive, but I strongly disagree. There is no need for any money to be involved. Many longstanding groups collect no fees. The value of the group lies in the experience, not in the cost.

## Food

A few groups meet over meals, or serve snacks. My concern would be that this might diffuse the clinical focus of the meeting, but I recognize that, depending on the group, this could have very minimal effect, if any.

## Contract

Only one of our interviewees was able to articulate a group contract, and that group took place within an agency setting. Confidentiality is often assumed, but too often little else is consciously explained or discussed. In forming a new group, I think it would be useful to spend the first meeting (or more) consciously and carefully defining the rules and agreements of the group, including how presentations are made, how feedback is given, guidelines for social contact, and how to raise and process issues in the group itself. For example, it might be helpful to have an agreement that group members do not discuss group dynamics outside of the meetings during social contacts. New members need to be informed about what the agreements are, which doesn't seem to happen very often. Many times, as one person said, it's just "Welcome to the group."

## Turnover

Dropouts can happen in any group. My sense is that this happens after a long period of dissatisfaction, with that person having many unvoiced or unaddressed complaints and unhappiness. Regular processing of this kind of material can often prevent dropout, although in some cases the person is in the wrong group and simply does not fit.

Most groups do have some attrition, and open spaces need to be filled if the group is to survive. New members can be brought in by any existing member, but perhaps a probationary period of three to six months would be a good idea, to see how the new person fits with the others.

## Social Contact

In most of the peer groups I know about, some of which were not included in the interviews, members are friends as well as colleagues, and have been socializing with each other for years before being in group together. While socializing outside of group meetings is discouraged or even proscribed in most therapy groups, this is not practical or even necessary in peer groups, provided that people don't form secret alliances and subgroups by discussing group issues.

My own experience is that social contact can enhance the feelings of closeness and safety in the group, but that sometimes unspoken and unaddressed group issues can be discussed outside of the group itself, in a way that compromises the integrity of the group.

## Leadership Functions

Although Goldberg (1981) suggests rotating leadership, and a couple of our groups did format themselves that way, it seems to me that this way of organizing defeats much of the purpose of being in a peer group. I think it's much more effective, and supportive of the members, for these functions to be shared among the membership at every meeting.

# Presentation

There are many different formats for presenting a case or an issue. I don't think it matters which one the group uses. The danger in this area, however, is of getting lost in facts and not focusing enough on feelings: What is it like to be in the room with the patient? What feelings come up among the peer group members listening to the presentation?

I think it is important for the presenter to follow up in the next meeting and give some reporting to the group about the impact of their feedback.

# Feedback / Safety and Trust

How feedback is given and what kinds of responses are useful can be discussed as part of the contract. Do we want to question the presenter? Do we want to simply make suggestions and say what we would do? How do we keep presenters from feeling criticized or even shamed? I think conscious choice about how the group wants to do this is better than not discussing it.

# Process

By *process* I mean that the group sets aside time on a regular basis, either a portion of every meeting or the entire meeting at periodic intervals, to discuss what goes on in the group itself. It may even be useful to say that process trumps presentation—any issue dealing with the group itself is more important and more urgent than a particular case. This might be the scariest, and the most difficult, aspect of group functioning. Many groups resist doing process, but I think it is crucial. Issues that go unvoiced and unaddressed are unlikely to simply go away, but more often will fester and grow, undermining the cohesion and longevity of the group. This is the time to bring up complaints, criticisms, or unhappiness with any aspect of group life. Conflicts between members can be addressed immediately, before they become ongoing resentments. Anything inhibiting or compromising optimal functioning can be examined and repaired.

# Conflict

I think it is inevitable that at some point in the life of every group, there will be some conflict between two or more members. If the group has been doing regular and consistent processing as described above, these conflicts will almost certainly be manageable, and will not threaten the existence of the group. Those members not directly involved in the controversy can help mediate and moderate the discussion until resolution is accomplished. The conflict may be countertransferential, in the sense that someone is triggering some personal historical issue in another member. It may be something more grounded in the present reality of how people are actually participating in the meetings. But whatever the issue, it must be addressed and not swept under the rug.

# A final word

From time to time, we hear of therapists who have crossed the line, lost their way, and gotten themselves into ethical or even legal trouble. It seems to me that this would be so much less likely to happen if that therapist were in some kind of peer supervision situation. I think that anyone presenting to a group regularly, even if he wasn't presenting his most questionable work, would find himself self-correcting those problematic behaviors that would lead to the kind of trouble that gets people sued, or even prosecuted.

While it is impractical to try to make this mandatory, I wish there were some way to promote this idea: that the very nature of private practice demands regular ongoing support from colleagues who understand the nature of the job, the pressures and difficulties of the task, the personal insight and self-awareness that the work itself requires. This support may also be available from a traditional supervisor, but that kind of relationship may be problematic for an experienced senior clinician. Peer supervision groups offer a wonderful solution.

# Appendix A—The Questionnaire

1. What is your professional background?
2. What is your theoretical orientation?
3. How long have you been in private practice?
4. How long have you been in the current peer group?
5. Have you been in other peer groups?
6. How did you find this group?
7. Did you know the people in the group before you joined?
8. What made you seek out such a group?
9. What is the makeup of the group?
10. Has there been much turnover?
11. How often and how long do you meet? Is that enough time?
12. Where do you meet?
13. Is there any kind of a contract?
14. How does the group normally begin?
15. Do you discuss your personal lives?
16. Do you socialize? How do you think that affects the functioning of the group?
17. Are there any fees involved?
18. Are people often absent? How does that affect the group?
19. What is the structure of a typical meeting?
20. Do you read papers/books and discuss them?
21. What kinds of issues usually get brought up?
22. Do the men function differently from the women?
23. Are you ever nervous about presenting a case?
24. Was there ever a case you didn't bring up because of concern about the group's reaction?
25. How often do you present a case?
26. What kinds of issues lead you to present a case?

27.    How do you process the feedback you get? How useful is the feedback? Is it ever confusing?

28.    Has the group ever told you that you shouldn't have done what you did?

29.    Do you ever notice a parallel process in the group when a case is being presented?

30.    How would you describe what you get from the group?

31.    What's missing from your group experience?

32.    How is a peer group different from a group with a leader?

33.    Do group members refer patients to each other? Is there anyone you wouldn't refer to?

34.    Has there ever been overt conflict? What was the nature of it? How are conflicts resolved?

35.    Is there anyone in the group you often disagree with?

36.    Is there anyone in the group you don't like?

37.    Has there ever been a crisis that threatened the existence of the group?

38.    What do you like best about the group?

39.    What do you like least about the group?

40.    Have you ever thought about leaving the group?

41.    Is there anything else about your experience that we haven't covered that you want to mention?

# REFERENCES

Akhurst, J., & Kelly, K. (2006). Peer group supervision as an adjunct to individual supervision: Optimising learning processes during psychologists' training. *Psychology Teaching Review, 12*(1), 3–15.

Allen, G. J., Szollos, S. J., & Williams, B. E. (1986). Doctoral students' comparative evaluations of best and worst psychotherapy supervision. *Professional Psychology: Research and Practice, 17*(2), 91–99.

Alonso, A. (1985). *The quiet profession: Supervisors of psychotherapy.* New York: Macmillan.

Alonso, A., & Rutan, J. S. (1988). Shame and guilt in psychotherapy supervision. *Psychotherapy: Theory, Research, Practice, Training, 25*(4), 576–581.

Altfeld, D. A., & Bernard, H. S. (1999). Experiential group psychotherapy supervision. *GROUP, 23*(1), 1–17.

Aronson, M. L. (1990). A group therapist's perspectives on the use of supervisory groups in the training of psychotherapists. *Psychoanalysis & Psychotherapy, 8*(1), 88–94.

Barnat, M. R. (1973). Student reactions to supervision: Quests for a contract. *Professional Psychology. 4*(1), 17–22.

Billow, R. M., & Mendelsohn, R. (1987). The peer supervisory group for psychoanalytic therapists. *GROUP, 11*(1), 35–46.

Bordin, E. S. (1983). Supervision in counseling: II. Contemporary models of supervision: A working alliance based model of supervision. *Counseling Psychologist, 11*(1), 35–42.

Brugger, T., Caesar, G., Frank, A., & Marty, S. (1962). Peer supervisor as a method of learning psychotherapy. *Comprehensive Psychiatry, 3*(1), 47–53.

Cohen, R. J., & DeBetz, B. (1977). Responsive supervision of the psychiatric resident and clinical psychology intern. *American Journal of Psychoanalysis, 37*(1), 51–64.

Counselman, E. F. (1991). Leadership in a long-term leaderless women's group. *Small Group Research, 22*(2), 240–257.

Counselman, E. F., & Gumpert, P. (1993). Psychotherapy supervision in small leader-led groups. *GROUP, 17*(1), 25–32.

Counselman, E. F., & Weber, R. L. (2004). Organizing and maintaining peer supervision groups. *International Journal of Group Psychotherapy, 54*(2), 125–143.

Cresci, M. B. (1996). How does supervision teach? Facilitating the supervisee's learning. *Psychoanalysis & Psychotherapy, 13*(1), 50–58.

Crick, P. (1991). Good supervision: On the experience of being supervised. *Psychoanalytic Psychotherapy, 5*(3), 235–245.

Doxsee, D. J., & Kivlighan, D. M. (1994). Hindering events in interpersonal relations groups for counselor trainees. *Journal of Counseling & Development, 72*(6), 621–626.

Emerson, S. (1996). Creating a safe place for growth in supervision. *Contemporary Family Therapy, 18*(3), 393–403.

Enyedy, K. C., Arcinue, F., Puri, N. N., Carter, J. W., Goodyear, R. K., & Getzelman, M. A. (2003). Hindering phenomena in group supervision: Implications for practice. *Professional Psychology: Research and Practice, 34*(3), 312–317.

Ettin, M. F. (1995). From one to another: Group consultation for group psychotherapy. *GROUP, 19*(1), 3–18.

Frawley-O'Dea, M. G. (1998). Revisiting the "teach/treat" boundary in psychoanalytic supervision: When the supervisee is or is not in concurrent treatment. *Journal of the American Academy of Psychoanalysis & Dynamic Psychiatry, 26*(4), 513–527.

Gill, S. (Ed). (2001). *The supervisory alliance: Facilitating the psychotherapist's learning experience.* Lanham, MD: Jason Aronson.

Gold, J. H. (2006). Why psychotherapy supervision is essential for mental health professionals. In *Psychotherapy supervision and consultation in clinical practice* (pp. 7–20). Lanham, MD: Jason Aronson.

Goldberg, C. (1981). The peer supervision group: An examination of its purpose and process. *GROUP, 5*(1), 27–40.

Gray, L. A., Ladany, N., Walker, J. A., & Ancis, J. R. (2001). Psychotherapy trainees' experience of counterproductive events in supervision. *Journal of Counseling Psychology, 48*(4), 371–383.

Hess, A. K. (1986). Unveiling the inner sanctum of psychotherapy supervision. *PsycCRITIQUES, 31*(12), 1005–1006.

Hess, A. K. (1997). The interpersonal approach to the supervision of psychotherapy. In C. E. Watkins Jr. (Ed.) *Handbook of psychotherapy supervision* (pp. 63–83). Hoboken, NJ: Wiley.

Hess, A. K. (1987). Psychotherapy supervision: Stages, Buber, and a theory of relationship. *Professional Psychology: Research and Practice, 18*(3), 251–259.

Hess, A. K., & Hess, K. A. (1983). Psychotherapy supervision: A survey of internship training practices. *Professional Psychology: Research and Practice, 14*(4), 504–513.

Hirsch, I. (1998). Discussion of Frawley-O'Dea and Sarnat: Emotional and interactional factors in the supervisory relationship. *Journal of the American Academy of Psychoanalysis & Dynamic Psychiatry, 26*(4), 545–552.

Hogan, R. A. (1964). Issues and approaches in supervision. *Psychotherapy: Theory, Research & Practice, 1*(3), 139–141.

Holloway, E. L., & Johnston, R. (1985). Group supervision: Widely practiced but poorly understood. *Counselor Education and Supervision, 24*(4), 332–340.

Hubble, M., Duncan, B., & Miller, S. (1999). *The heart and soul of change.* Washington, DC: American Psychological Association.

Hunt, W. (1981). The use of the countertransference in psychotherapy supervision. *Journal of the American Academy of Psychoanalysis & Dynamic Psychiatry, 9*(3), 361–373.

Hunt, W., & Issacharoff, A. (1975). History and analysis of a leaderless group of professional therapists. *American Journal of Psychiatry, 132*(11), 1164–1167.

Issacharoff, A., & Hunt, W. (1977). Observations on group process in a leaderless group of professional therapists. *GROUP, 1*(3), 162–171.

Itzhaky, H., & Itzhaky, T. (1996). The therapy–supervision dialectic. *Clinical Social Work Journal, 24*(1), 77–88.

Kassan, L. D. (1996). *Shrink Rap: Sixty Psychotherapists Discuss Their Work, Their Lives, and the State of Their Field.* Northvale, NJ: Jason Aronson.

Kassan, L. D. (1999). *Second opinions: Sixty psychotherapy patients evaluate their therapists.* Northvale, NJ: Jason Aronson.

Kassan, L. D. (2007). *Who could we ask? The gestalt therapy of Michael Kriegsfeld.* New York: iUniverse.

Kassan, L. D. (2008). Encounters in the waiting room. *Annals of the American Psychotherapy Association, 14*(3), 20–23.

Kennard, B. D., Stewart, S. M., & Gluck, M. R. (1987). The supervision relationship: Variables contributing to positive versus negative experiences. *Professional Psychology: Research and Practice, 18*(2), 172–175.

Kline, F. M. (1972). Dynamics of a leaderless group. *International Journal of Group Psychotherapy, 22*(2), 234–242.

Kline, F. M. (1974). Terminating a leaderless group. *International Journal of Group Psychotherapy. 24*(4), 452–459.

Kozlowska, K., Nunn, K., & Cousens, P. (1997a). Training in psychiatry: An examination of trainee perceptions. Part 1. *Australian and New Zealand Journal of Psychiatry, 31*(5), 628–640.

Kozlowska, K., Nunn, K., & Cousens, P. (1997b). Adverse experiences in psychiatric training. Part 2. *Australian and New Zealand Journal of Psychiatry, 31*(5), 641–652.

Lachmann, F. M. (2003). Supervision: The devil is in the details. *Psychoanalytic Dialogues, 13*(3), 341–353.

Ladany, N. (2007). Does psychotherapy training matter? Maybe not. *Psychotherapy: Theory, Research, Practice, Training, 44*(4), 392–396.

Ladany, N., Friedlander, M. L., & Nelson, M. L. (2005a). *Critical events in psychotherapy supervision: An interpersonal approach.* Washington, DC: American Psychological Association.

Ladany, N., Friedlander, M. L., & Nelson, M. L. (2005b). Negotiating role conflicts: If it were easy, it wouldn't be called supervision. In *Critical events in psychotherapy supervision: An interpersonal approach.* (pp. 79–97). Washington, DC: American Psychological Association.

Ladany, N., Friedlander, M. L., & Nelson, M. L. (2005c). Working through countertransference: When supervision is needed. In *Critical events in psychotherapy supervision: An interpersonal approach* (pp. 99-126). Washington, DC: American Psychological Association.

Ladany, N., Hill, C. E., Corbett, M. M., & Nutt, E. A. (1996). Nature, extent, and importance of what psychotherapy trainees do not disclose to their supervisors. *Journal of Counseling Psychology, 43*(1), 10–24.

Langs, R. (1994). Combining supervision with empowered psychotherapy. *Contemporary Psychoanalysis, 30*(1), 25–47.

Lewis, G. J., Greenburg, S. L., & Hatch, D. B. (1988). Peer consultation groups for psychologists in private practice: A national survey. *Professional Psychology: Research and Practice, 19*(1), 81–86.

McNeill, B. W., & Worthen, V. (1989). The parallel process in psychotherapy supervision. *Professional Psychology: Research and Practice, 20*(5), 329–333.

Mintz, E. (1968). Group supervision for mature therapists. *Journal of Group Psychoanalysis & Process, 1*(2), 63–70.

Mintz, E. (1983). Gestalt approaches to supervision. *Gestalt Journal, 6*(1), 17–27.

Montgomery, A. G. (1978). Issues in therapist training and supervision. *Psychology: A Journal of Human Behavior, 15*(2), 28–36.

Moskowitz, S. A., & Rupert, P. A. (1983). Conflict resolution within the supervisory relationship. *Professional Psychology: Research and Practice, 14*(5), 632–641.

Moss, E. (1995). Group supervision: Focus on countertransference. *International Journal of Group Psychotherapy, 45*(4), 537–548.

Murray, M. E. (1974). Attitudes toward supervision in professional clinical training. *Psychotherapy: Theory, Research & Practice., 11*(3), 293–312.

Nelson, G. L. (1978). Psychotherapy supervision from the trainee's point of view: A survey of preferences. *Professional Psychology, 9*(4), 539–550.

Nelson, M. L., & Friedlander, M. L. (2001). A close look at conflictual supervisory relationships: The trainee's perspective. *Journal of Counseling Psychology, 48*(4), 384–395.

Nestler, E. J. (1990). The case of double supervision: A resident's perspective on common problems in psychotherapy supervision. *Academic Psychiatry, 14*(3), 129–136.

Nobler, H. (1980). A peer group for the therapists. *International Journal of Group Psychotherapy, 30*, 51–61.

Norman, J., & Salomonsson, B. (2005). 'Weaving thoughts': A method for presenting and commenting psychoanalytic case material in a peer group. *International Journal of Psychoanalysis, 86*(5), 1281–1298.

Nunberg, H., & Federa, P. (1962), *Minutes of the Vienna Psychoanalytic Society*, vol. 1. New York: International Universities Press.

O'Connor, B. P. (2000). Reasons for less than ideal psychotherapy supervision. *Clinical Supervisor, 19*(2), 173–183.

Ogren, M., Apelman, A., & Klawitter, M. (2001). The group in psychotherapy supervision. *Clinical Supervisor, 20*(2), 147–175.

Ogren, M., & Sundin, E. C. (2007). Experiences of the group format in psychotherapy supervision. *Clinical Supervisor, 25*(1-2), 69–82.

Overholser, J. C. (1991). The Socratic method as a technique in psychotherapy supervision. *Professional Psychology: Research and Practice, 22*(1), 68–74.

Overholser, J. C. (2004). The four pillars of psychotherapy supervision. *Clinical Supervisor, 23*(1), 1–13.

Pate, L. A., & Wolff, T. K. (1990). Supervision: The residents' perspective. *Academic Psychiatry, 14*(3), 122–128.

Peake, T. H., Nussbaum, B. D., & Tindell, S. D. (2002). Clinical and counseling supervision references: Trends and needs. *Psychotherapy: Theory, Research, Practice, Training, 39*(1), 114–125.

Phillips, G. L., & Kanter, C. N. (1984). Mutuality in psychotherapy supervision. *Psychotherapy: Theory, Research, Practice, Training, 21*(2), 178–183.

Pines, M. (1987). Review of *The Quiet Profession—Supervisors of Psychotherapy. Group Analysis, 20*(4), 381.

Prieto, L. R. (1996). Group supervision: Still widely practiced but poorly understood. *Counselor Education and Supervision, 35*(4), 295–307.

Rabinowitz, F. E., Heppner, P. P., & Roehlke, H. J. (1986). Descriptive study of process and outcome variables of supervision over time. *Journal of Counseling Psychology, 33*, 292–300.

Robiner, W. N., & Schofield, W. (1990). References on supervision in clinical and counseling psychology. *Professional Psychology: Research and Practice, 21*(4), 297–312.

Rosenthal, L. (2005). Group supervision of groups: A modern analytic perspective. *Modern Psychoanalysis, 30*(2), 167–184.

Salvendy, J. T. (1993). Control and power in supervision. *International Journal of Group Psychotherapy, 43*(3), 363–376.

Sarnat, J. E. (1998). Rethinking the role of regressive experience in psychoanalytic supervision. *Journal of the American Academy of Psychoanalysis & Dynamic Psychiatry, 26*(4), 529–543.

Schröder, T. A., & Davis, J. D. (2004). Therapists' experience of difficulty in practice. *Psychotherapy Research, 14*(3), 328–345.

Searles, H. F. (1955). The informational value of the supervisor's emotional experiences. *Psychiatry, 18*, 135–146.

Shanfield, S. B., Matthews, K. L., & Hetherly, V. (1993). What do excellent psychotherapy supervisors do? *American Journal of Psychiatry, 150*(7), 1081–1084.

Shanfield, S. B., Mohl, P. C., Matthews, K. L., & Hetherly, V. (1992). Quantitative assessment of the behavior of psychotherapy supervisors. *American Journal of Psychiatry, 149*(3), 352–357.

Shatan, C. F., Brody, B., & Ghent, E. R. (1962). Countertransference: Its reflection in the process of peer-group supervision. *International Journal of Group Psychotherapy, 12*(3), 335–346.

Shultz, P. P., & Stoeffler, V. R. (1986). Group supervision in a retreat setting: The continuing process of becoming a psychotherapist. *Group Analysis, 19*(3), 223–234.

Teitelbaum, S. H. (1990). Aspects of the contract in psychotherapy supervision. *Psychoanalysis & Psychotherapy, 8*(1), 95–98.

Steinhelber, J., Patterson, V., Cliffe, K., & LeGoullon, M. (1984). An investigation of some relationships between psychotherapy supervision and patient change. *Journal of Clinical Psychology, 40*(6), 1346–1353.

Talbot, N. L. (1995). Unearthing shame in the supervisory experience. *American Journal of Psychotherapy, 49*(3), 338–349.

Teitelbaum, S. (1995). The changing scene in psychoanalytic supervision. *Psychoanalysis & Psychotherapy, 12*(2), 183–192.

Todd, W. E., & Pine, I. (1968). Peer supervision of individual psychotherapy. *American Journal of Psychiatry, 125*(6), 780–784.

Tyler, J. D., Sloan, L. L., & King, A. R. (2000). Psychotherapy supervision practices of academic faculty: A national survey. *Psychotherapy: Theory, Research, Practice, Training, 37*(1), 98–101.

Wallace, E., & Alonso, A. (1994). Privacy versus disclosure in psychotherapy supervision. In S. E. Greben & R. Ruskin (Eds). *Clinical perspectives on psychotherapy supervision* (pp. 211–230). Washington, DC: American Psychiatric Association.

Watkins, C. E. (1990). Development of the psychotherapy supervisor. *Psychotherapy: Theory, Research, Practice, Training, 27*(4), 553–560.

Watkins, C. E. (1992). Reflections on the preparation of psychotherapy supervisors. *Journal of Clinical Psychology, 48*(1), 145–147.

Watkins, C. E. (1995a). Psychotherapy supervisor development: On musings, models, and metaphor. *Journal of Psychotherapy Practice & Research, 4*(2), 150–158.

Watkins, C. E. (1995b). Pathological attachment styles in psychotherapy supervision. *Psychotherapy: Theory, Research, Practice, Training, 32*(2), 333–340.

Watkins, C. E. (1995c). Psychotherapy supervision in the 1990s: Some observations and reflections. *American Journal of Psychotherapy, 49*(4), 568–581.

Watkins, C. E. (1996). On demoralization and awe in psychotherapy supervision. *Clinical Supervisor, 14*(1), 139–148.

Watkins, C. E. (1997). The ineffective psychotherapy supervisor: Some reflections about bad behaviors, poor process, and offensive outcomes. *Clinical Supervisor, 16*(1), 163–180.

Weaks, D. (2002). Unlocking the secrets of 'good supervision': A phenomenological exploration of experienced counsellors' perceptions of good supervision. *Counselling & Psychotherapy Research, 2*(1), 33–39.

Webb, A., & Wheeler, S. (1998). How honest do counsellors dare to be in the
supervisory relationship?: An exploratory study. *British Journal of Guidance & Counselling, 26*(4), 509–524.

West, W. (2003). The culture of psychotherapy supervision. *Counselling & Psychotherapy Research, 3*(2), 123–127.

Whitman, S. M. (2001). Teaching residents to use supervision effectively. *Academic Psychiatry, 25*(3), 143–147.

Whitman, S. M., & Jacobs, E. G. (1998). Responsibilities of the psychotherapy
supervisor. *American Journal of Psychotherapy, 52*(2), 166–175.

Winnicott, D. W. (1965). *The maturational processes and the facilitating environment.* New York: International Universities Press.

Worthen, V., & McNeill, B. W. (1996). A phenomenological investigation of
"good" supervision events. *Journal of Counseling Psychology, 43*(1), 25–
34.

Worthington, E. L. (1987). Changes in supervision as counselors and supervisors gain experience: A review. *Professional Psychology: Research and
Practice, 18*(3), 189–208.

Yerushalmi, H. (1992a). Psychoanalytic supervision and the need to be alone.
*Psychotherapy: Theory, Research, Practice, Training, 29*(2), 262–268.

Yerushalmi, H. (1992b). On the concealment of the interpersonal therapeutic
reality in the course of supervision. *Psychotherapy: Theory, Research,
Practice, Training, 29*(3), 438–446.

Yerushalmi, H. (1994). A call for change of emphasis in psychodynamic supervision. *Psychotherapy: Theory, Research, Practice, Training, 31*(1), 137–
145.

Yerushalmi, H. (1999a). The roles of group supervision of supervision. *Psychoanalytic Psychology, 16*(3), 426–447.

Yerushalmi, H. (1999b). Mutual influences in supervision. *Contemporary Psychoanalysis, 35*(3), 415–436.

Yogev, S., & Pion, G. M. (1984). Do supervisors modify psychotherapy supervision according to supervisees' levels of experience? *Psychotherapy:
Theory, Research, Practice, Training, 21*(2), 206–208.

Yourman, D. B. (2003) Trainee disclosure in psychotherapy supervision: The
impact of shame. *Journal of Clinical Psychology, 59*(5), 601–609.

Yourman, D. B. & Farber, B. A. (1996). Nondisclosure and distortion in psychotherapy supervision. *Psychotherapy: Theory, Research, Practice, Training,
33*(4), 567–575.

# Index

# About the Author

Lee D. Kassan is a licensed psychoanalyst, licensed mental health counselor, and certified group psychotherapist in private practice in New York City since 1980. He has been associate editor of the professional journal *GROUP* since 2001, and serves on the Board of Directors of the Eastern Group Psychotherapy Society. He trained at the American Institute for Psychotherapy and Psychoanalysis in New York.

He is also author of *Who Could We Ask? The Gestalt Therapy of Michael Kriegsfeld* (2007), *Second Opinions: Sixty Psychotherapy Patients Evaluate Their Therapists* (1999), and *Shrink Rap: Sixty Psychotherapists Discuss Their Work, Their Lives, and the State of Their Field* (1996), and a coauthor of *Genius Revisited: High IQ Children Grown Up* (1993).

You can visit his website at www.leekassan.com.